TECHNICAL

MAGNETIC

RESONANCE

IMAGING

TECHNICAL
MAGNETIC
RESONANCE
IMAGING

John A. Markisz, MD, PhD
Associate Professor of Radiology
Cornell University Medical College
New York, New York

Associate Attending Radiologist
Chief, Division of Magnetic Resonance
The New York Hospital
New York, New York

Michael Aquilia, RT
Chief Technologist, Magnetic Resonance Imaging
Cornell University Medical Center
New York, New York

APPLETON & LANGE
Stamford, Connecticut

Copyright © 1996 by Appleton & Lange
A Simon & Schuster Company

96 97 98 99 00 / 10 9 8 7 6 5 4 3 2 1

Prentice Hall International (UK) Limited, *London*
Prentice Hall of Australia Pty. Limited, *Sydney*
Prentice Hall Canada, Inc., *Toronto*
Prentice Hall Hispanoamericana, S.A., *Mexico*
Prentice Hall of India Private Limited, *New Delhi*
Prentice Hall of Japan, Inc., *Tokyo*
Simon & Schuster Asia Pte. Ltd., *Singapore*
Editora Prentice Hall do Brasil Ltda., *Rio de Janeiro*
Prentice Hall, *Upper Saddle River, New Jersey*

Library of Congress Cataloging-in-Publication Data
Technical magnetic resonance imaging / John A. Markisz, Michael G. Aquilia.
    Includes bibliographical references.
    ISBN 0-8385-8836-0 (pbk. : alk. paper)
    1. Magnetic resonance imaging. 2. Nuclear magnetic resonance
spectroscopy. I. Markisz, John A. II. Aquilia, Michael G.
    [DNLM: 1. Magnetic Resonance Imaging. 2. Magnetic Resonance
Imaging—atlases.   WN 185 T255 1996]
RC78.7.N83T43 1996
616.07'548—dc20
DNLM/DLC   96-1712
for Library of Congress   CIP

ISBN 0-8385-8836-0

9 780838 588369   90000

Acquisitions Editor: Jane Licht
Production Editor: Sondra Greenfield
Designer: Mary Skudlarek

PRINTED IN THE UNITED STATES OF AMERICA

To Our Families:

Adele, Andy, Bob, Sue, Chris, Katie

— John A. Markisz

Kim, Gisele, Charlie, Michael, Natalie

— Michael Aquilia

CONTENTS

PREFACE

Although there have been many important developments in diagnostic imaging over the past several decades, none has been as great a departure from conventional radiology as the introduction of magnetic resonance imaging (MRI). Now accepted as a basic imaging tool, MRI is used in almost every field of medicine. MRI therefore has affected not only technologists and radiologists, but health-care workers in every discipline of medicine as well.

We wrote this text to provide those directly involved with MRI, technologists and radiologists, with a practical discussion of the technical aspects involved in actually performing MRI. We discuss all the techniques encountered in patient handling, scanning, and positioning. We explain the relationships of the various scanning parameters and effects on image quality and imaging time as well as provide a basic explanation of fundamental principles involved in MRI.

Precautions and contraindications to imaging have never been as challenging. There are a vast array of new terms and concepts to be understood and to be explained to patients. This new modality has an enormous array of capabilities ranging from images, to angiography, to evaluation of cardiac motion and joint mobility. New uses are continually being developed, with functional imaging and spectroscopy appearing on the horizon.

We hope that our book will enable technologists currently working in the field to increase their technical knowledge and provide information to assist in improving performance. We also hope that our book will acquaint residents and physicians with the practical aspects involved in scanning and protocoling various examinations. Finally, we hope that this book will give health-care professionals in all areas of medicine who deal with patients having MR examinations a basic understanding of the practical side of the procedure, so that professionals will be better able to explain the procedure to their patients and answer their questions more effectively.

ACKNOWLEDGMENTS

....

The authors are grateful and wish to express their sincere appreciation to

- The technical staffs of the Division of Magnetic Resonance of Cornell University Medical College and The New York Hospital, for their assistance in obtaining much of the material that went into the development of this text: Richard Fischer, Sangjoon Park, Edna Hong, Chul Lee, Carol Green, John Crespo, and Kim Iarrucci.

- Drs. Patrick T. Cahill and R. James R. Knowles, for their development and testing of many of the pulse sequences, applications, and quality assurance procedures described in this manual.

- Dr. Mary Ann Payne for her constant support and encouragement.

- James Zaput and James McCormack, of General Electric Medical Systems, for sharing their technical insights with us.

- Ms. Jane Licht of Appleton & Lange, whose patience and perseverance were appreciated by the authors and ultimately resulted in the production of this text.

TECHNICAL

MAGNETIC

RESONANCE

IMAGING

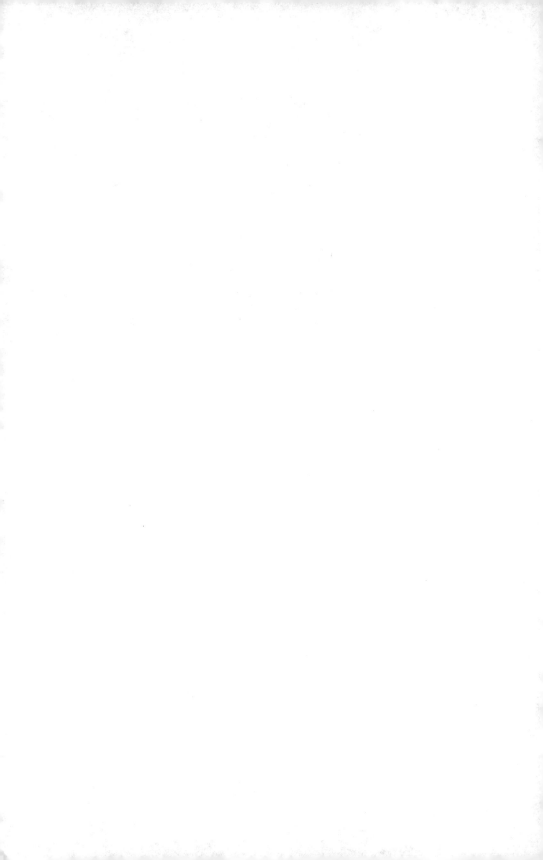

CHAPTER ONE

MAGNETISM AND MAGNETIC PROPERTIES OF MATTER

A basic understanding of the principles of magnetism and magnetic resonance is necessary in order to understand how MRI units operate, how to obtain the best possible studies, and how to determine when the system is malfunctioning. Since an in-depth treatment of the physics underlying magnetic resonance and magnetic resonance imaging is beyond the scope of this text, what follows is an elementary description of the fundamental principles of magnetic resonance and their applications to imaging. A bibliography is supplied in Appendix A on page 253 for those interested in pursuing topics in greater detail.

MAGNETISM

The concept of magnetism dates to the sixth century B.C., when the ancient Greeks discovered that a naturally occurring magnet, the mineral lodestone (called magnetite after the district Magnesia where it was found), would attract pieces of iron. Plato wrote that Socrates described how magnetite would support a chain of iron rings, one above another, by magnetic attraction.

The Roman philosopher Lucretius Carus described magnetic repulsion as well as attraction. Magnetic attraction was explained on the basis that the magnetite had small hooks on it, and the iron had small rings on it that caught on the hooks. The invention of the magnetic compass is attributed to the Chinese mathematician Shen Kua (1030–1093), who described its use on land in the eleventh century A.D. Arab sailors were known to use the magnetic compass for navigation on the seas in the twelfth century. The first reference to its use by European sailors came in the mid-thirteenth century. Ardent scientific research in magnetism began in the latter half of the nineteenth century and has continued to the present day.

The magnetic properties we observe in nature, in materials that we call magnets, arise from unpaired spinning electrons in the atoms. This is a different source than the magnetic forces that are used in magnetic resonance imaging, but the magnetic effect is the same. Natural occurring magnets, of which lodestone is the most common example, are usually formed of oxides of iron and can be found as crystals, rocks, beach sand, meteorites, and emery. The largest deposits of natural magnets are found in northern Sweden, and the most powerful magnetic rocks are found in Siberia and on the island of Elba. These natural or permanent magnets are important industrially, being found in speakers, generators, motors, and telephone receivers, as well as on refrigerator doors. In addition to natural magnets, science has found methods of creating large magnetic fields by using electrical currents and by using superconducting materials at very low temperatures.

Central to the understanding of magnetism is a force field that exists around every magnet. Each magnet has two opposite poles, called north and south poles because of the way in which they will align in the Earth's magnetic field. The strength of a magnetic field depends upon the strength of the force field around each magnet. The lines of the force field can be observed by placing a magnet on a piece of paper and carefully sprinkling iron filings on the paper around the magnet. Magnets do not have to be in contact to attract a piece of iron, and this action-at-a-distance is due to the presence of the magnetic field surrounding each magnet. When two magnets are brought close to

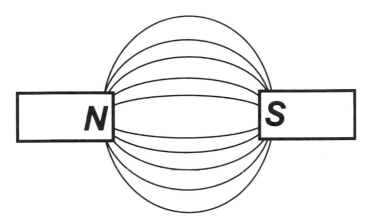

Figure 1–1. When two opposite magnetic poles are brought close together they will attract one another. This figure shows the lines of force between opposite poles.

each other, the alignment of the poles will determine what happens. Opposite poles attract (Figure 1–1), while like poles repel (Figure 1–2). The farther away one is from a magnet, the weaker is the effect of field. A magnet can be represented by a vector, or arrow, with the head of the arrow representing one pole of the magnet and the tail of the arrow representing the other pole. The direction of the arrow indicates the direction of the magnetic field (Figure 1–3). (The way in which the strength of the magnetic field will vary at different distances around a magnetic resonance imaging system can be seen in Figures 5–3 and 5–4.)

For centuries, the strength of magnetic fields was measured in units called **gauss**. The unit, abbreviated as G, was named in honor of Carl Friedrich Gauss (1777–1855), a German physicist and mathematician. Gauss was a child prodigy who taught himself reading and arithmetic by the time he was three, and during his lifetime made major contributions to many areas of mathematics and physics, including magnetism. The magnetic field of the earth varies between 0.3 and 0.7 G, depending upon how far one is from the North Pole, and averages approximately 0.5 G. During the middle and later parts of this century, scientists have been able to generate very strong

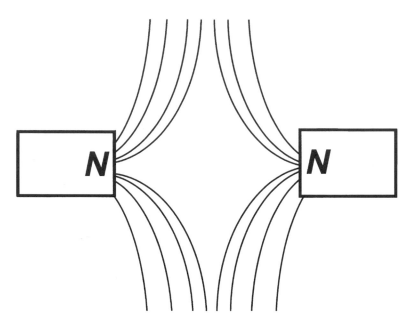

Figure 1–2.   When similar magnetic poles are brought together, there is a repulsion, with the magnetic lines of force attempting to push the magnets apart.

magnetic fields, well over 100,000 G. MRI units are currently approved for field strengths up to 15,000 G.

Since these large numbers become relatively awkward to use, a larger unit, the **tesla,** was proposed. One tesla (abbreviated as T) is equal to 10,000 gauss. This unit was named in honor of Nikola Tesla (1856–1943), a rather eccentric Croatian physicist who emigrated to the United States in 1884. At the age of 5 he built a waterwheel that did not have any paddles, and in later life he used this machine as the model for his unique bladeless turbine engine. Tesla worked briefly for Thomas Edison; however, a lifelong feud between the two soon developed. Their rivalry reached such proportions that their refusal to share the 1915 Nobel Prize for Physics resulted in neither one obtaining it. Tesla patented an alternating-current motor, which was bought by George Westinghouse and became the basis for Westinghouse products. Tesla also did a significant amount of

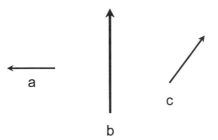

Figure 1–3.   Magnetic fields can be represented by arrows, with the head of the arrow symbolizing the north magnetic pole and the tail of the arrow symbolizing the south magnetic pole. These arrows are actually vectors: they have size and direction. Part a represents a small horizontal magnetic field, with the north pole directed to the left; part b represents a large vertical magnetic field, with the north magnetic pole directed upwards; part c illustrates a medium-sized magnetic field directed at an angle, as shown.

research in magnetic fields, including inventing the principle of the rotary magnetic field, which eventually permitted hydroelectric power to be transmitted from Niagara Falls. He was considered quite peculiar in his day, believing in seances to contact the spirit world, proposing to build a vacuum tube under the Atlantic to transport mail, and a rotary platform around the equator to encircle the Earth. He spoke about having plans for "secret weapons" and a death and disintegrator ray, and although he never published them, all of his papers were confiscated by the U.S. military upon his death and remain classified to this day. In fact, a letter written in 1945 by an Army officer referring to the location of the papers was classified as top secret under the Espionage Act and was not declassified until 1980. His biography makes very interesting reading.[1, 2]

FERROMAGNETISM, PARAMAGNETISM, AND DIAMAGNETISM

One method of classifying materials is by their magnetic properties. They can be divided into ferromagnetic, paramagnetic, and diamagnetic substances.

Ferromagnetic materials (*ferro* from the Latin term for iron) are inherently magnetic, whether or not they are in a magnetic field. These are the naturally occurring magnets, such as the mineral lodestone or magnetite. These substances, usually containing iron, are called permanent magnets. Ferromagnetic materials are composed of many small permanent magnets, all aligned in the same direction (Figure 1–4). They can be made to lose their magnetism if they are heated above certain temperatures (the Curie temperature, different for each substance), at which point these small magnets become randomly arranged and their magnetic properties cancel one another. The magnetic properties of a permanent magnet can also be destroyed by applying a stronger magnetic field in the opposite direction for a long period of time.

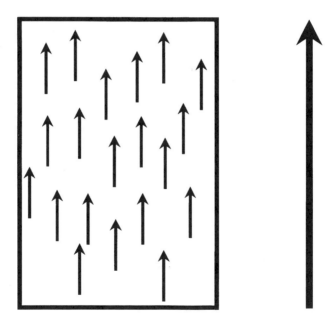

Figure 1–4.   Ferromagnetic substances are composed of tiny atomic magnets, each oriented in the same direction. The combination of these small magnets produces a large overall magnetic effect.

Paramagnetic substances have no naturally occurring magnetic properties until they are placed within a magnetic field. They are thought to contain small magnetic dipoles, which are randomly arranged and do not produce a magnetic field (Figure 1–5A). When they are placed within a magnetic field, these dipoles line up with the field, acquire an induced magnetization, and are strongly attracted to the magnetic field (Figure 1–5B). Gadolinium is an example of a paramagnetic substance. When placed in a magnetic field, gadolinium atoms become strongly magnetic, interacting with the applied field.

Diamagnetic materials are substances that are actually repelled from a magnetic field. Like paramagnetic substances,

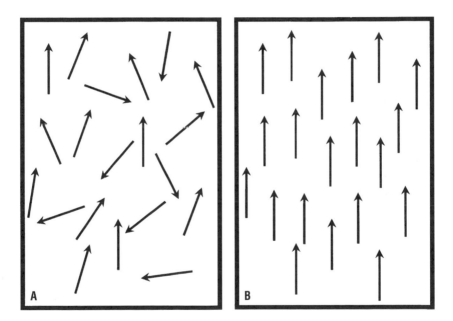

Figure 1–5. (A) Paramagnetic materials are composed of tiny atomic magnets. Their orientation is completely random, however, so that the magnetic effect of each small magnet is cancelled out and the overall effect is a nonmagnetic material. (B) When placed in an applied magnetic field, these small magnets will line up with the field and the paramagnetic material acquires an induced magnetization.

they have no inherent magnetic properties unless they are placed within a magnetic field. The repulsive force is very weak when compared to ferromagnetism and paramagnetism and will rarely be noticed unless carefully arranged experiments are performed. Gold, copper, lead, and water are examples of diamagnetic materials.

ELECTROMAGNETS

In addition to permanent magnets, a second type of magnet is an **electromagnet**. As the name implies, this type of magnet utilizes an electric current. The British physicist Michael Faraday found that an electromagnet could be produced by winding a coil of wire around an iron core and passing an electric current through the wire. The system acts as a magnet only as long as the current is flowing. The field disappears once the current is stopped, so that the electromagnet has the advantage of being able to produce a magnetic field on demand, turning it on and off at will. When it is operational, an electromagnet requires a constant source of electric current. When used as the basis for a magnetic resonance imaging system, the need for continual electric power can add considerably to the cost of the operation.

An electric current is technically defined as an electric charge in motion. It is a type of energy. The most common type of electric current, and the only practical example, involves electrons moving through a wire. This type of energy is what runs almost every aspect of our everyday life. As the electrons move through the wire, they move fairly freely, but there is some resistance to the flow. This resistance is caused by the electrons colliding with the atoms in the wire, which can slow them down and result in a loss of energy. As the temperature of the wire becomes lower, the resistance becomes less and the electrons lose less energy. As the temperature is lowered past a certain point for many metals, the resistance to the flow of electrons disappears completely, and the metal is said to be a superconductor.

SUPERCONDUCTIVITY

Superconductivity is a phenomenon which requires extremely low temperatures. It was discovered in 1911 that many metals have a transition point temperature, ranging from between 1 and 10°Kelvin (°K) above absolute zero (0°K). Below this temperature, these metals will lose almost all resistance to the flow of an electric current. Since the magnetic-field strength set up by current flowing through a coil is inversely proportional to the resistance in the wire, the lower the resistance is, the higher will be the magnetic field generated. Therefore, if a metal has almost no electrical resistance, it can be used to generate very high magnetic fields. Liquid helium, which has a boiling point of 4.2°K (−269°C, −452°F), is required in order to achieve these temperatures. If the helium vapor is pumped off, the temperature of the liquid helium can be reduced even further, to 1°K. Normal liquid helium behaves like typical liquids; however, a second type of liquid helium, called liquid helium II, can be formed below 2°K. This material is an extraordinary substance, sometimes called a fourth state of matter, which has the peculiar ability to climb up the walls of the container and spill over the top.

When a coil of metal is cooled to these low temperatures, electrical current can move freely through it with essentially no resistance at all. The superconducting wires used in MRI systems are usually composed of alloys of niobium and titanium, which become superconducting below 10°K (−263°C or −441°F). If a small amount of current is placed in a superconducting system, it will not lose any energy and can flow indefinitely, as long as the coil is maintained at the low temperature. This flowing current will produce very high magnetic fields. One advantage of a superconducting magnet is that a small amount of current has to be introduced into the system only once. There is no need for a continuous electrical supply in order to preserve the magnetic field. One disadvantage is that once the field is established, there is no way to turn it off unless the temperature is allowed to increase. Since cooling the system down to the appropriate temperature and reestablishing a homogeneous magnetic field takes several weeks, the temperature of the superconducting magnet is never intentionally permitted to increase. The cost of maintaining sufficient liquid helium to keep the system at a low temperature was once an economic consideration. Many units had to be refilled every two weeks or less. Newer, more efficient systems, however, now require refilling with liquid helium only four to five times a year.

Quenching

Keeping a superconducting magnet at extremely cold temperatures is essential for proper operation. On rare occasions there may be a slight temperature increase, enough to lose the superconducting properties of the metal in the magnet. If this occurs, the system effectively becomes resistive, producing large quantities of heat, and the liquid helium begins to boil off. This process is called **quenching**. If the quenching is planned, for hardware changes or necessary maintenance, the process will be controlled and the boil-off will be slow. If, however, it occurs accidentally, there will be a very rapid boil-off of the cryogens (liquid helium and liquid nitrogen). Even though helium and nitrogen are not poisonous gases, they can force all of the oxygen out of the magnet room, introducing the potential for suffocating anyone trapped in the room. Superconducting magnets contain powerful exhaust vents and oxygen monitors to check on oxygen levels, just in case of an accidental quench. In order to be absolutely sure that oxygen is not being pushed out of a room by cryogens being boiled off, these oxygen monitors will sound an alarm when there has been a decrease of only a small amount of oxygen. Normal oxygen content of the air is 20%, and the oxygen monitor alarms will sound when the oxygen level has decreased to only 18%.

MAGNETIC PROPERTIES OF MATTER

The smallest part of any element is an atom. Atoms are composed of spinning particles, which are in turn composed of electrical charges. The center of an atom, called the nucleus, is composed in part of spinning positive charges, called protons, and spinning neutral particles, called neutrons. Spinning or moving electrical charges will create a magnetic field. Protons will therefore behave like small magnets.

As mentioned before, magnetic fields are vector quantities and can be represented by arrows. These arrows have both size and direction; that is, they point in a certain way. By convention, the head of the arrow represents the north pole of the magnet and the tail of the arrow represents the south magnetic pole. In the nucleus, protons usually tend to pair up, with oppositely aligned particles pairing up so that their magnetic properties cancel each other out. Unpaired protons will produce a net magnetic moment, causing the nucleus to behave like a small magnet. The hydrogen nucleus consists of a single proton, which is spinning on its axis, just as the earth does. As it spins, it sets up a magnetic field and behaves like a small magnet (Figure 1–6).

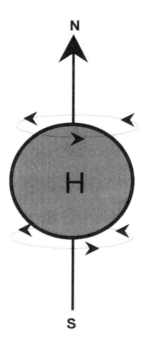

Figure 1–6. The spinning proton in the hydrogen nucleus produces a magnetic field and behaves as if it were a tiny magnet. It can be represented by a vector, as can any magnetic field.

The positively charged nucleus is surrounded by negatively charged electrons, which can be considered to be moving around the nucleus like planets orbiting the sun. For the purposes of magnetic resonance, only the positively charged nucleus is important, since the field created by the electrons is too weak to have an effect under the conditions employed in MRI. (Electron spin resonance does exist and is employed by chemists and physicists for other purposes, but it does not affect MRI.)

The spinning positive charges, or protons, in the nucleus create a magnetic field. In most atoms, which are composed of many protons, the magnetic fields caused by each proton will be arranged in opposite directions so that they cancel out or balance each other, and no net magnetic effects will be observed. In some atoms, however, there will not be any magnetic balance, resulting in a small atomic magnet. The hydrogen atom, which contains only one proton in its nucleus, is the most common and most abundant of these atomic magnets. Hydrogen atoms are used in magnetic resonance imaging for two reasons: first, the magnetic field set up by the spinning proton in the nucleus of the hydrogen atom is stronger than in most other atoms; and second, hydrogen atoms are the most common atoms in living tissue, comprising over 99% of all atoms in the body. For these reasons, the signal established by hydrogen atoms during an MRI scan is stronger than could be obtained by any other type of atom.

Consider for a moment the behavior of a compass used for determining direction. A compass is composed of a small magnet balanced on a thin rod so that it is free to rotate. In the Earth's magnetic field, one end of the magnet will always rotate so that it is pointing north, no matter how we turn the compass. The nucleus of a freely rotating hydrogen atom will behave in exactly the same way when placed in a magnetic field. The magnetic field of the hydrogen nucleus is so weak that it is not affected by the magnetic field of the Earth, and it will only be influenced by a very strong magnetic field. The magnetic fields used in imaging are between 6,000 and 30,000 times stronger than the magnetic field of the Earth. Under normal conditions the small atomic magnets are oriented in random directions. When placed in a strong magnetic field, however, these magnets will line up in the direction of the field, just as the needle of a compass lines up in the magnetic field of the Earth.

POINTS TO PONDER

- Spinning or moving electrical charges will create a magnetic field.

- The nucleus (center) of a hydrogen atom contains a single spinning proton (positively charged particle).

- It is the magnetic field of the hydrogen nucleus that is utilized in magnetic resonance imaging.

- Magnetic fields of magnets arise from unpaired electrons of the atoms.

- Magnets have opposite poles: north and south.

- Units of magnetic field strength are gauss (G) and tesla (T).

- 10,000 gauss = 1 tesla. The Earth's magnetic field is 0.5 G. MRI systems range from 0.3 to 1.5 T.

- Ferromagnetic materials are intrinsically magnetic, naturally occurring, most often containing iron ores.

- Paramagnetic materials are materials that do not exhibit magnetic properties unless placed in a magnetic field.

- Diamagnetic materials are repelled by magnetic fields; however, the force of repulsion is relatively weak.

- Electromagnets produce a magnetic field by using an electric current to flow through coils of wire.

- Superconductivity is the absence of resistance to the flow of an electric current in a metal.

- Superconducting magnets use liquid helium to produce the low temperatures needed to attain the superconducting state.

- An electric current flowing in a superconducting coil will produce an extremely high magnetic field.

REFERENCES

1.   Cheney M. *Tesla, Man Out of Time.* New York: Barnes & Noble Books; 1993.
2.   Martin TC. *The Inventions, Research, and Writings of Nikola Tesla,* 2nd ed. New York: Barnes & Noble Books; 1992.

CHAPTER TWO

IMAGES AND IMAGE QUALITY

Since medical images are used to make diagnoses, we strive to obtain the clearest and most well-defined picture possible. The amount of detail that we can distinguish in any picture is called the **resolution** of an image. It is usually measured in terms of how close together two lines can be placed and still be seen as two separate lines. Everyone has experienced taking photographs with different degrees of resolution, whether they realize it or not. Motion and distance are two factors that affect the resolution of a normal photograph, and, as we shall see later, can also affect MR images. If the subject or the camera is moving, the image will be blurred and details will not be well visualized. A photograph of a distant mountain will not have sufficient resolution to allow us to distinguish between two leaves on a tree, or possibly even two trees, but a photo of trees in the backyard might allow us to see individual leaves on the trees. In imaging the same type of problem occurs, and decisions have to be made about how we want to evaluate the medical problem: do we want an overview, where one can see a large area, in which structures are relatively small but we can see entire organ systems, or do we want to concentrate on a small part of the anatomy and increase the detail so that we can view even very small structures for smaller but still significant pathological changes?

The resolution of an MR image depends upon many factors. In order to better understand them, it is important to realize what an image is composed of. Figure 2–1A is a photograph of a head. The image is clear and appears to be quite smooth. If we take a small area of that image, indicated by the white rectangle, and magnify it five times, we see that our supposedly smooth picture is actually composed of a large number of small boxes (Figure 2–1B), each a different shade of gray. These boxes that make up the image are called **pixels**. The smaller each of these pixels is, the higher the resolution of our image and the clearer it appears to our eyes. Figure 2–2A is a cross-sectional view of an imaging phantom with the left-to-right distance covered by 128 pixels, while Figure 2–2B is the exact same section; however, 512 pixels, each one quarter of the size, were used to cover the same distance. The increased clarity of the second image demonstrates that the smaller the pixel is, the higher is the resolution. In an MR image, the number of pixels used in each dimension is referred to as the **matrix** size. The higher the matrix size, the smaller the size of each pixel and the greater is the detail that can be visualized. Every image that is looked at can be thought of as having two directions. Sometimes these directions can be referred to as up and down and left and right (as when viewing a picture); sometimes they are called horizontal and vertical; a mathematician might call these directions the x-axis and the y-axis. For reasons that will be explained in Chapter 4, the directions of an MR image are referred to as the **phase-encoding direction** and the **frequency-encoding direction**. These directions are interchangeable, and are often switched by the MR operator in order to minimize or eliminate artifacts. The number of pixels used in the phase-encoding direction is usually given first. A matrix size of 128 by 256 indicates that the distance in the phase-encoding direction was broken into 128 equal parts, while the distance of the frequency-encoding direction was divided into 256 equal parts.

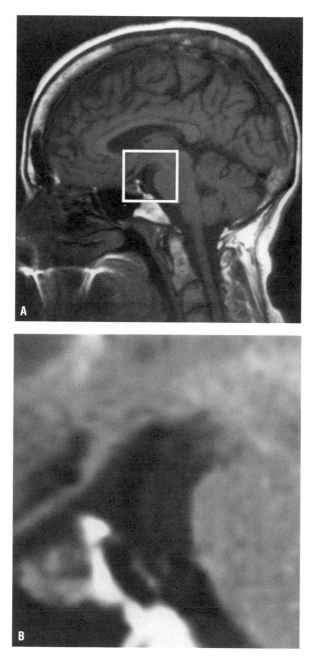

Figure 2–1.   (A) Sagittal image of the head. (B) The part of the image in the white box in A magnified five times. Note that the individual pixels are visible in the magnified image.

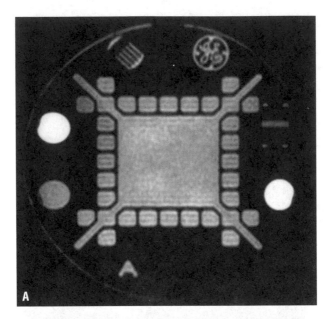

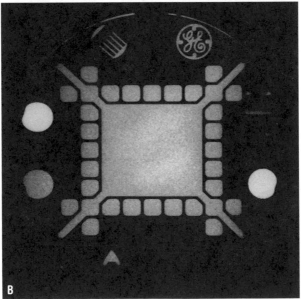

Figure 2–2. (A) View of a phantom at a 128-by-256 matrix. (B) Same phantom image as in A but acquired with a 512-by-512 matrix. Note how much clearer the image is with smaller pixels. Four signal averages and 10-mm-slice thickness increase total signal within each pixel to minimize effect of noise (see Figure 2–10).

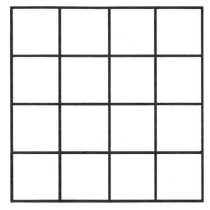

Figure 2–3. An image is composed of pixels, which are a series of boxes as shown here. In an actual image, each pixel will be a different color (colored images) or a different shade of gray (black-and-white images).

In an MR image it is important to remember that although the image itself is two-dimensional (Figure 2–3), with no thickness, it actually represents an anatomic section that does have a thickness to it. The pixels that form the image are two-dimensional rectangles, but actually represent a three-dimensional box, where the third dimension is the thickness of the slice. These three-dimensional boxes are called **voxels** (Figure 2–4). The terms pixel and voxel are often incorrectly used interchangeably; however, it is a common occurrence and the distinction should be clear. When we are referring to an image, which is flat and has no thickness, we are dealing with pixels. Each MR image represents a thin slice of anatomic tissue, which has a certain thickness and is actually composed of many thousands of voxels (little volumes). When the image is printed, it is flat and is composed of the same number of two-dimensional pixels, where each pixel represents a voxel in the actual tissue.

THE IMAGE MATRIX

Figure 2–5 shows examples of different simple matrix types. Matrices do not have to be even along each side (axis) and the individual pixels can be either square or rectangular. The pictures

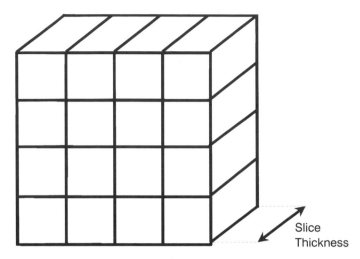

Slice
Thickness

Figure 2–4.   In an MRI image, in which a slice or section of anatomy is imaged, there is a thickness of the slice, which means that the two-dimensional pixels of the image are actually representations of three-dimensional voxels of the actual slice. Voxels, then, are actually pixels with a thickness.

in Figure 2–6 demonstrate how the different matrix sizes affect the quality of an image. If we attempt to image a black cross, shown in Figure 2–6A, in the simplest type of matrix, one pixel (Figure 2–6B), we see in Figure 2–6C that part of the pixel is filled with the black of the image, but part is also not filled with anything. This averages out to a dark gray box (Figure 2–6D), a very low resolution picture that looks nothing like the actual image. As the number of pixels increases, and therefore the size of each pixel gets smaller, the shape of the image produced becomes closer to that of the actual object (Figures 2–7A–C). In a 4-by-4 matrix, none of the pixels are completely filled, but some are three-quarters filled and some are half filled, so the image begins to resemble a cross. In an 8-by-4 matrix (Figures 2–8A–C), the central pixels are completely filled and appear black, and other pixels are partially filled and the image is closer to reality. In an 8-by-8 matrix (Figures 2–9A–C), the pixels are small enough so that we get an accurate representation of what we are imaging.

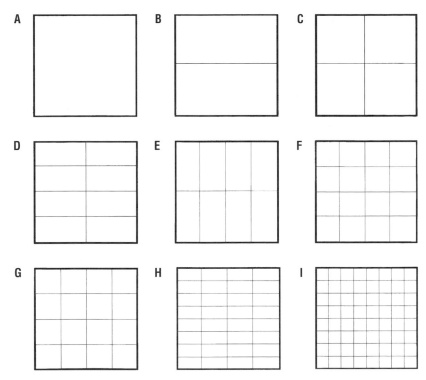

Figure 2–5. Pixels can be large or small, square or rectangular, as illustrated in the above examples.

It would appear quite logical, then, that to obtain the best-quality images, we should always strive for smaller and smaller pixel sizes, which would give us the highest resolution possible. Unfortunately, practical considerations do not make things so simple. The first factor to be considered in the production of the MR image is the signal obtained. As will be discussed in Chapter 3, the strength of the signal ultimately depends upon the size of a quantity called the **transverse magnetization**. The amount of signal produced from a particular voxel depends upon how much tissue is in it. If the pixel size is very small, the amount of signal coming from it will be too small, resulting in a poor image quality.

The greater the amount of tissue, the stronger the signal emanating from the voxel. The thicker the slice or the smaller

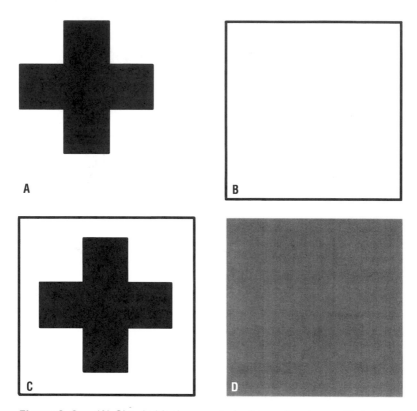

Figure 2–6.   (A) Simple black cross to be imaged, using multiple techniques. (B) Using one large pixel to form the image. (C) The cross fits within the image, but does not fill it. (D) The color of the cross plus the lack of color of the empty space is averaged to give the pixel a uniform gray intensity. This is the final image using a one-pixel matrix.

the matrix size, the larger the volume of the voxel, the larger the amount of tissue in the voxel, and therefore the stronger the signal. Unfortunately, increasing the size of the voxel decreases the resolution, so a compromise must be made on voxel size, which is determined by matrix size and slice thickness. Additional factors affecting the signal strength will be discussed in the following chapters.

The hardware and software currently available has practical limits, so that a matrix size of 512 by 512 pixels is currently the largest that can be used. A second consideration is the time

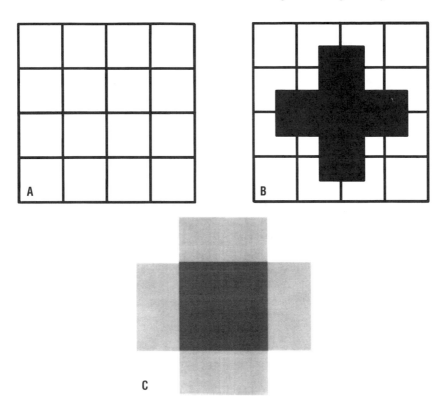

Figure 2–7. (A) Using a 4-by-4 pixel matrix, with the same overall size as before. (B) The cross overlaps multiple pixels. It fills three quarters of the four central pixels and fills one quarter of the middle two pixels in each outside row. (C) The three-quarter-filled pixels are darker than the outside one-quarter-filled pixels, producing the final image, which begins to resemble a cross.

that the examination will take. The higher the matrix size (the greater the number of pixels), the longer the examination takes. The total imaging time for a routine spin-echo sequence can be given by the equation:

$$\textbf{time} = \textbf{(P.E. matrix size)} \times \textbf{TR} \times \textbf{N}_{ex} / \textbf{1000}$$

where the time is given in seconds, P.E. matrix size is the number of pixels in the phase-encoding direction, TR is the repetition time (see Chapter 4), and N_{ex} is the number of signal averages used. This will be discussed in detail in Chapters 6 and 7.

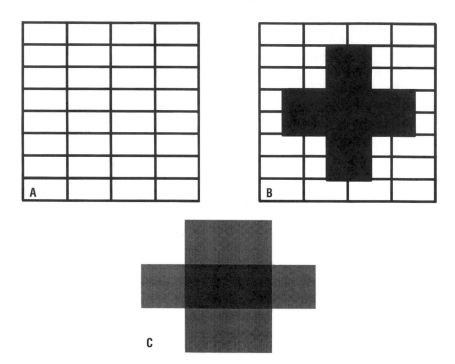

Figure 2–8.   (A) Using an 8-by-4 matrix with rectangular pixels to form the image. (B) The four central pixels are completely filled by the cross and the twelve adjacent pixels are half filled. (C) The resulting image is somewhat skewed because of the use of rectangular pixels, but they are closer in color and resemble a cross.

A series of images obtained with a 256-by-256 matrix would take twice as long to obtain as the same images with a 128-by-256 matrix. We strive to obtain the best images possible, even though longer imaging times might produce higher resolution images, but increasing the imaging time will sometimes have the opposite effect, producing poor images because of the patients' inability to remain motionless for long periods of time. Increased scanning time will also decrease the number of patients that are able to obtain an examination.

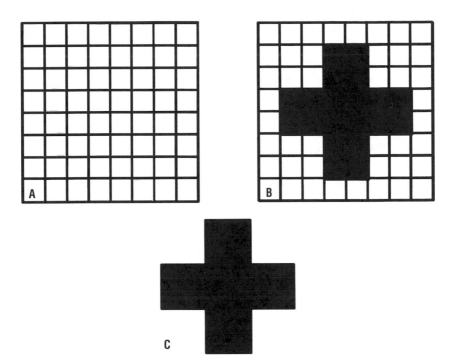

Figure 2–9. (A) Using a matrix composed of 8-by-8 square pixels to form the image. (B) The cross fits over the pixels and all pixels are either completely filled or completely empty. (C) The use of a larger number of smaller pixels produces an exact replica of the original image.

NOISE AND SIGNAL-TO-NOISE RATIO

The **intensity** of each pixel (or actually each voxel)—that is, how bright or how dark it is—depends upon how much radiofrequency (rf) signal is detected within the voxel. A large amount of signal will make the pixel bright, while if little or no signal is obtained, the pixel will be dark. A special problem arises in situations where there is interference or a break in the rf shield, or if very large matrix values (producing very small voxels) are used. This problem is referred to as **noise**, which is signal generated by unrelated sources that is attributed to random signal within the voxels. If the voxels have sufficient signal, we do not notice this extraneous signal that is added to the true signal. However, if the voxel is too small, this extra signal from outside sources can make a significant difference in what the image looks like and the resultant image is termed **noisy**.

During the production of the MR image (which we will discuss in Chapter 4), the material in each voxel produces a radiofrequency (rf) signal, which is picked up and analyzed by the computer. If the voxel is large, it will produce a lot of signal; if it is small, it will produce a lesser signal. Unfortunately, the tissue within the voxel is not the only source of rf signal. There are unavoidable sources of stray rf signal called **noise**, or background signal coming from the equipment, the tissues of the patient, and outside sources such as radio and television signals. These stray signals can be added into a given voxel. If the voxel is large, there is a strong signal coming from it and the effect of the noise is negligible. If the voxel is made too small, however, the stray noise has a significant effect and the quality of the image and results in a noisy, or degraded, image. The size of the voxel can be increased by increasing the slice thickness, or by decreasing the matrix size (using a smaller number of pixels).

To observe the impact of noise, consider images shown in Figures 2–10A and 2–10B. These images are divided into thousands of voxels, with each voxel eventually represented by a pixel in our final image. Figure 2–10A was obtained using a 256-by-128 matrix (32,768 pixels) and Figure 2–10B with a 512-by-512 matrix (262,144 pixels). The voxels used in obtaining Figure 2–10A were eight times larger than those in Figure 2–10B. The additional signal covers up the effects of stray noise, improving the appearance of the image.

The quality of the MR signal is measured by the **signal-to-noise ratio (SNR)**. Mathematically, this is simply a measurement of the intensity of the signal of the tissue divided by the intensity of the noise (usually measured as intensity in a region without any tissue). The higher the signal-to-noise ratio, the less noisy and the better the quality of the image obtained. In addition to the larger voxel size discussed above, other factors that will increase the SNR are an increased field of view, a decreased sampling bandwidth, increased spacing between slices and an increased number of signal averages, all of which

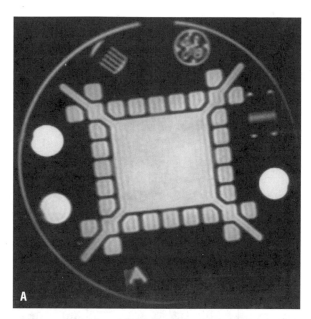

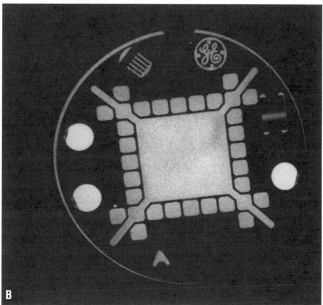

Figure 2–10.   (A) A 256-by-128 matrix was used to obtain this image, which is relatively uniform in signal quality. (B) Using a 512-by-512 matrix results in a less homogeneous image because the signal from each pixel is less, and the effect of random noise is greater.

will be discussed later. Also inherent in the determination of the SNR is the field strength of the magnet. The higher the field strength of the magnetic resonance imaging system, the higher will be the SNR. This is one reason that many manufacturers have pushed toward using higher field strengths. Increasing static magnetic field strength increases available signal because at the higher field strength there are more nuclei aligned with the field. This results in more nuclei interacting with the rf pulse that ultimately produces the signal from the tissue. With all other factors constant, approximate relative SNR values for a 0.5 T system is 6; for a 1.0 T system, 12; and for a 1.5 T system, 22.

SLICE THICKNESS

The thickness of the slices will affect both the quality of the images and the quality of the interpretations. The thicker the slice, the larger will be the size of the voxel, and the more signal will be contained within it. This combination will give the appearance of a high-quality image, with an inherently higher SNR. Although the images will be more pleasing to the eye if the slice thickness is increased, too thick a slice may conceal important clinical information. Consider a 5-mm-thick lesion in the liver. If a 1-cm- (10-mm-) thick section is used in imaging, for example, half of the voxel would contain the lesion and the other half would contain normal liver tissue. Depending upon how different the lesion signal was from normal liver, the lesion might be obscured by the normal tissue that is imaged with it in the same voxel. Figure 2–11 illustrates how slice thickness can affect the final image.

CONTRAST

The final important factor in determining the overall quality of an image is **contrast**: the relative ability to distinguish two adjacent objects in an image due to differences in their brightness. A total lack of contrast would be found in the proverbial picture of a polar bear in a snowstorm. Maximum contrast would be

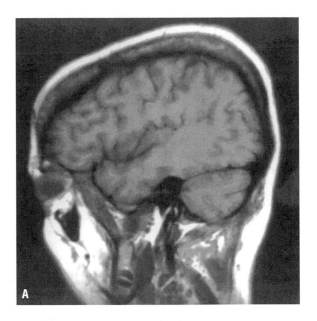

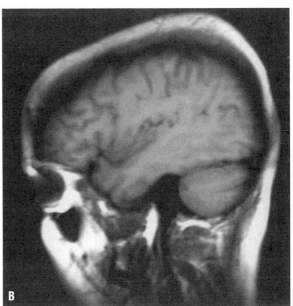

Figure 2–11.   (A) A 3-mm-thick slice is quite sharp in delineating objects. (B) A 10-mm-thick slice through the same area blends small objects together so that the resolution is decreased.

achieved by viewing a totally black ball on an absolutely white background. A difference in contrast is thus essential to our definition of resolution, the ability to distinguish objects in an image. In an MR image, brightness is directly proportional to signal intensity, so that the contrast of two objects can be measured in terms of differences in their signal intensity. Unlike computerized axial tomography (CT) or other imaging modalities utilizing radiation, there is no absolute value of signal intensity in MRI. All pixels are normalized to the average maximum signal intensity, so that numerical values of intensity can vary significantly from scan to scan and magnet to magnet. Measuring relative signal intensity in adjacent voxels A and B will lead to a definition of contrast as:

$$\textbf{contrast} = (I_a - I_b)/I_0$$

where I_a and I_b are signal intensities in adjacent pixels and I_0 is the average maximum signal intensity.

POINTS TO PONDER

- Resolution is the smallest distance between two objects that can clearly be distinguished.

- Images are composed of tiny boxes called pixels. The smaller that the pixels are, the higher is the resolution of the image.

- A matrix indicates the number of pixels along each axis in an image.

- Voxels are three-dimensional boxes, or small volumes, which compose part of the image.

- Imaging time depends upon the matrix size in the phase-encoding dimension, the repetition time (TR), and the number of signal averages (N_{ex}).

- The intensity of a pixel depends upon how much signal is detected within a voxel.

CHAPTER THREE

PRINCIPLES OF MAGNETIC RESONANCE

MAGNETIC RESONANCE

The discovery of magnetic resonance of nuclei was made in 1946 by two Americans, each working independently.[1, 2] Swiss-born Felix Bloch of Stanford and Edward Mills Purcell of Harvard had worked together during World War II on an anti-radar project for the government. After the war they returned to their respective laboratories, where they independently and almost simultaneously discovered the phenomenon of nuclear magnetic resonance. They were jointly awarded the Nobel Prize for Physics in 1952.

The concept was first termed NMR, for nuclear magnetic resonance, and was quickly developed into an important spectroscopic method for chemists, physicists, and biologists to use to determine the structure of complex organic molecules. This method developed into a routine laboratory procedure during the 1950s and 1960s. Significant advances in applying this technique were made during this time, utilizing not only chemicals, but biological tissues as well. In 1971, Dr. Raymond Damadian reported the use of NMR signals for the detection of tumors.[3]

In 1973, Dr. Paul Lauterbur, at Stony Brook, published the first report on using signals from nuclear magnetic resonance to produce images.[4]

As mentioned previously, hydrogen atoms are the most important type of atom for magnetic resonance imaging, because they are so abundant and because they possess a high magnetic moment. Since an atomic magnet has two poles, north and south, it is sometimes referred to as a magnetic dipole (Figure 3–1). The hydrogen atoms in the tissues within the body can be divided into two types: those that are so tightly bound to other atoms that they will not be able to move in a magnetic field, and those that can move when placed in a magnetic field. This last group are referred to as **mobile protons** and constitute the majority of the hydrogen atoms in the body. Only these mobile protons are involved in magnetic resonance.

Under normal conditions, without an outside magnetic field, the magnetic vectors representing hydrogen nuclei are randomly oriented, as illustrated in Figure 3–2. When the hydrogen nuclei are placed in a strong magnetic field, they will align themselves parallel to the direction of the field, either pointing in the same direction or, for those with higher energy, pointing in the opposite direction (Figure 3–3). There is a slight difference in energy in the two cases: if the atoms are aligned so that they are pointing in the same direction as the applied field, they will have a slightly lower energy than atoms that are aligned opposite to the field (Figure 3–4). There is always a slightly greater number pointing with the

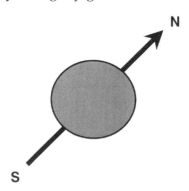

Figure 3–1.   Each hydrogen nucleus behaves as if it were a small magnet, with a north and a south magnetic pole.

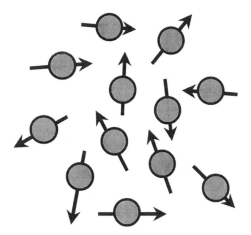

Figure 3–2. Atoms, each behaving as a small magnet, are randomly oriented under normal conditions.

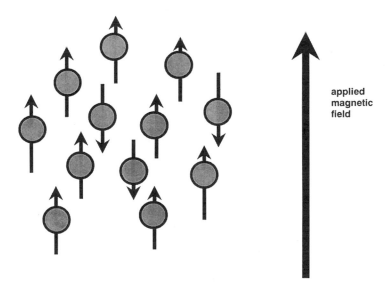

applied
magnetic
field

Figure 3–3. In an applied magnetic field, these small magnets align themselves in the direction of the field, with more pointing with the field than against it.

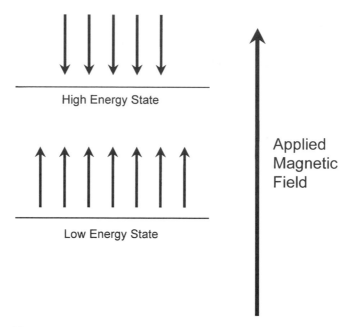

Figure 3–4. Atoms that align their magnetic fields in the same direction as the applied magnetic field have a slightly lower energy than those atoms that align their fields opposite to the applied field. Under normal conditions there are always a few more atoms in the lower energy state than in the high energy state.

field (lower energy state) than pointing opposite to it (slightly higher energy state), but all the atoms are aligned parallel to the applied field. At 1.5 T, for every million hydrogen atoms, there are only about 5 more atoms in the low energy state (pointing with the field) than there are in the high energy state (pointing opposite to the field). Atoms can move from the low energy state to the high energy state if they can acquire additional energy. This energy is a definite, fixed amount, which depends upon the magnetic field strength. It is referred to as the Larmor energy, which will be discussed below (Figure 3–5).

Once the mobile protons have lined up in the magnetic field, they will remain that way, just as a magnetic needle in a compass will remain pointing north. The needle in a compass will not move unless something is done to it. In order to disturb the equilibrium, a force must be applied or energy supplied to

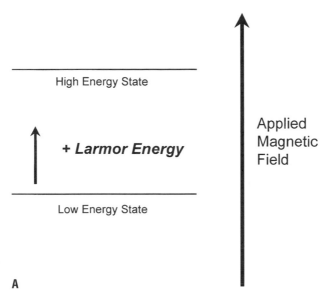

Figure 3–5A.   An atom that is aligned with the applied magnetic field can absorb only a specific amount of energy, which corresponds to the Larmor frequency.

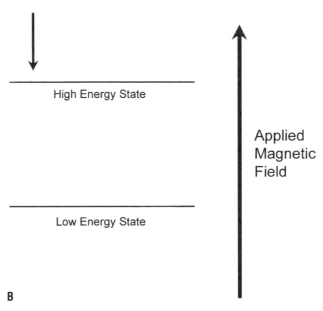

Figure 3–5B.   After absorbing this energy, the atom jumps up into the higher energy state, in which its magnetic vector has been reversed so that it is aligned opposite to the applied field.

the system, or it will not change. The needle will move, for example, if kinetic energy is added in the form of a push from someone's finger or if a force field of a magnet is brought alongside of the compass.

In order to alter the equilibrium of the hydrogen nuclei that are aligned in the applied magnetic field, electromagnetic energy is used. Electromagnetic energy is a type of radiation that has both electric and magnetic components and ranges from the very-high-energy gamma rays to the low-energy radio waves. Table 3–1 lists different types of electromagnetic radiation with their associated physical properties. The various types of waves are characterized by different frequencies. Gamma rays, X-rays, and ultraviolet radiation are high-energy, high-frequency forms of

TABLE 3–1. SPECTRUM OF ELECTROMAGNETIC RADIATION

Radiation	Energy (eV)*	Frequency (MHz)	Wavelength (cm)	
Gamma rays	$>10^6$	$>10^{14}$	$>10^{-10}$	Emitted by radioactive nuclei
X-rays	$10-10^5$	$10^{10}-10^{14}$	$10^{-6}-10^{-10}$	Emitted when high energy electrons collide with metals
Ultraviolet rays	10	10^9	10^{-5}	From solar radiation; screened out by ozone layer; dangerous
Visible light	1	10^8	$10^{-3}-10^{-4}$	Violet, indigo, blue, green, yellow, orange, red; the combination produces white light
Infrared rays	$10^{-2}-10^{-3}$	10^7	$10^{-2}-10^{-3}$	Widely used for heating
Radar waves	10^{-5}	10^5	1	Low energy radiation used in location of distant objects; used by bats in echolocation
Microwaves	10^{-4}	10^4	10	Low energy level; used in telecommunications since they can carry more information than radio waves
TV waves	10^{-7}	10^2	10^2	Present system of electronic image transmission proposed by A. A. Campbell-Swinton of Scotland in 1908
Radiowaves	$10^{-7}-10^{-9}$	$1-10^2$	10^2-10^4	First used for wireless communications by Marconi in 1895

* electron volts

electromagnetic radiation. These types of radiation are referred to as ionizing radiation because of their potential to ionize material within cells, especially DNA, which can be harmful to biological systems. Visible light is also a form of electromagnetic energy that is of lower, nonharmful energy. Each color has a particular frequency, which can interact with the human retina and be interpreted by the brain as an image of a particular color. Radiowaves are at the low-energy, low-frequency end of the electromagnetic spectrum. It is radiowaves that are used in magnetic resonance imaging. Frequencies that are within the radiowave range are called radiofrequencies and are abbreviated rf.

In addition to spinning on its axis, in a manner similar to the Earth rotating on its axis, each spinning proton also precesses. Figure 3–6 illustrates the precession that every hydrogen atom undergoes in a magnetic field. Precession is a wobbly type of motion, analogous to a spinning top that is losing energy and beginning to follow a cone-shaped path, rather than spinning straight up. This means that the precessing atoms are not really aligned exactly in the direction of the

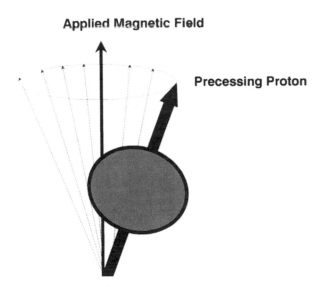

Applied Magnetic Field

Precessing Proton

Figure 3–6. In addition to spinning on its axis, as does the Earth, in a magnetic field the atomic magnet also precesses, outlining a cone-shaped path.

applied field, but are angled slightly off of it. In a given magnetic field, all hydrogen atoms precess at the same frequency, called the **Larmor frequency**. This frequency depends upon the field strength of the magnet, and is given by the Larmor equation:

$$\mu = \gamma B_0$$

where μ is the Larmor frequency, γ is a constant for each atom called the gyromagnetic ratio (42.58 MHz/T for hydrogen), and B_0 is the applied field strength. The Larmor frequency for hydrogen corresponds to the radiofrequency range in all imaging systems; in a 1.5 T magnetic field it is 63 MHz. Most MR imaging systems operate between 0.15 T and 1.5 T, which correspond to 6.3 MHz and 63 MHz, respectively. In the electromagnetic spectrum (Table 3–1), these frequencies correspond to the upper FM or lower CB radio bands through to the lower VHF television bands. Since these frequencies are continuously being broadcast and will interfere with the MR images, the magnet rooms must be rf-shielded to keep these unwanted radiowaves away from the vicinity of the magnet.

The hydrogen nuclei that are placed into the magnetic field are aligned with the field and are simultaneously precessing around the axis of the magnetic field. They can be "pushed" out of alignment by "hitting" the atoms with electromagnetic energy. Only certain radiofrequencies, the Larmor frequency, will work at each magnetic field strength. For example, at an external magnetic field strength of 1.5 T, rf waves of only 63 MHz will interact, while at 0.5 T only 21 MHz rf energy can be used. In terms of the high and low energy states, when a nucleus in the low energy state (aligned in the same direction as the field) is exposed to energy that is exactly enough to move it into the next-highest energy state, it will absorb the energy and move into the high energy state (aligned in the opposite direction as the field) (Figure 3–5A). A short pulse of radiowaves of the proper frequency is directed at the aligned hydrogen atoms, which knocks them out of alignment (Figure 3–7). When the rf pulse is terminated, the protons begin to move back into alignment with the external magnetic field (Figure 3–8).

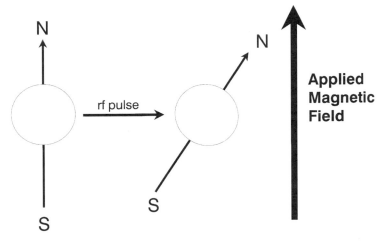

Figure 3–7.   After the rf pulse introduces energy of the proper frequency (Larmor equation), the atoms are knocked out of alignment.

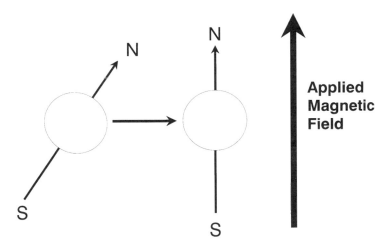

Figure 3–8.   After the pulse is turned off, the atoms attempt to regain their equilibrium state.

The term **resonance** in physics usually refers to a situation where only a certain specific energy will cause a change, most often a major change. If a tuning fork set for a definite note is struck, it will begin to sound the note. Any other tuning fork in the

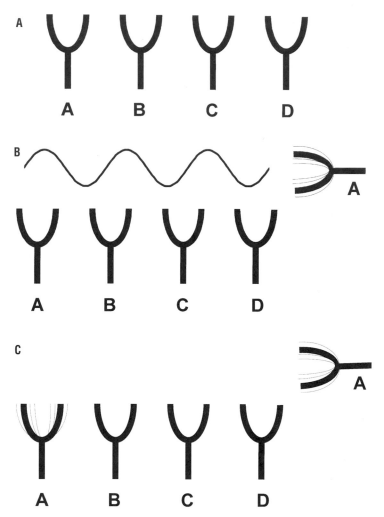

Figure 3–9. (A) Tuning forks are constructed so that they will vibrate only at a particular frequency, which corresponds to a certain note of the scale (A, B, C, D, etc.). (B) If a tuning fork of a particular frequency (for example, corresponding to the note A) is struck, it will send out energy waves of the frequency of note A. (C) These waves can interact with another tuning fork only if it is of the exact same frequency and start the other fork vibrating as well. In this example only the tuning fork that vibrates with the note A begins vibrating when another A is sounded. This phenomenon is one example of resonance.

room that is set for the exact same note will undergo resonance and begin to sound, even though it has not been touched (Figure 3–9). Crystalline goblets can also have a resonant frequency at which they vibrate, usually corresponding to a frequency of a high-pitched sound. Should an opera singer hit a high note corresponding to that resonant frequency, the goblet will pick up energy from the sound, begin to vibrate, and may eventually shatter.

The resonant frequency in magnetic resonance is the Larmor frequency. Only energy corresponding exactly to the Larmor frequency can be absorbed by the nuclei in the magnetic field. When energy of that frequency is supplied, major changes occur.

Only when rf energy corresponding to the Larmor frequency is provided to the precessing nuclei can the atoms absorb the energy and resonance occur. The energy is provided in the form of a pulse of rf radiation of the proper Larmor frequency. The extra energy causes the atoms to precess at a greater angle, so the magnetic vector associated with the atom tips farther away from the applied field. When enough energy is added so that the atom precesses through an angle of 90°, it is called a 90° pulse (Figure 3–10). When it has flipped through a 90° angle, it is in the *xy*, or transverse, plane, and all of the atoms are precessing "in phase," which is another way of saying that they are precessing together.

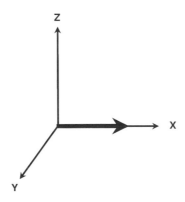

Figure 3–10.   When enough energy is added to flip the magnetic vector 90°, the vector is in the *xy*, or transverse, plane.

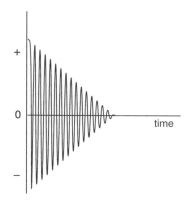

Figure 3–11. The rf signal obtained by the receiver coil continually decreases with time, in the form of a decaying sinusoidal wave, and is called free induction decay (FID).

After the rf pulse has been stopped, all of the nuclei begin to attempt to get back to their equilibrium position, which is (1) aligning with the applied magnetic field and (2) attaining the normal rate of precession. In order to return to the equilibrium state, the rf energy that had been absorbed by the atoms is released. This energy decays rapidly and is referred to as free induction decay (FID). The transverse magnetization in the xy plane induces an alternating current in the rf receiver coil. Since the components in the xy plane diminish continually after the rf pulse has been turned off, the signal received by the rf receiver coil decreases continuously with time. The shape of this signal can be described as a decaying sinusoidal wave (Figure 3–11).

Returning to equilibrium is called **relaxation** and can be thought of as a two-step process, with each step having its own relaxation time. A relaxation time is a measure of the time needed to regain equilibrium: mathematically it is the time necessary for a system to regain $1/e$ (e is the natural base), or approximately 63% of its original value. First, realignment with the applied field is called **longitudinal**, or **T1, relaxation** and is controlled by a time constant referred to as T1. The T1, or longitudinal, relaxation time is the time that it takes for 63% of the nuclei to realign with the external magnetic field. In T1 relaxation, after the magnetic moment is flipped 90° by the application of a pulse of rf energy, the pulse is turned off. This is followed by a gradual return to

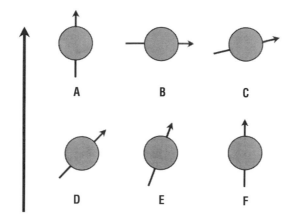

Figure 3–12. T1 relaxation. (A) Initially the magnetic field of the atom is aligned with the applied magnetic field. (B) The rf pulse is then applied and the magnetic field has been rotated by 90°. After the cessation of the rf pulse, the overall magnetic vector begins to return to its equilibrium position (C–E) until in F it has regained an equilibrium position.

equilibrium, as the magnetic vector eventually returns to its equilibrium position along the z axis (Figure 3–12).

The second type of relaxation, which occurs simultaneously with the T1 relaxation, is called the **T2**, or **transverse, relaxation**. This process is more difficult to describe, as it involves the rate of precession of the different nuclei. Just after the rf pulse is applied, all of the nuclei are precessing together, in phase, at the exact same rate. Once the rf pulse is stopped, each atom finds itself in a *slightly* different magnetic environment, since the atoms surrounding atom A will be different in type and position from those surrounding atom B. Because there is a slight difference in their magnetic environments, atom A and atom B start to precess at different rates. They are no longer in phase, with those in higher fields precessing faster and those in lower fields precessing more slowly. As their motions become more and more random, the magnetization in the transverse plane is lost (Figure 3–13). The time constant controlling how fast this process occurs is called the T2, or transverse, relaxation time. As with the T1 values, the T2 value is the time it takes for 63% of the nuclei to be out of phase with each other. The transverse relaxation occurs much more

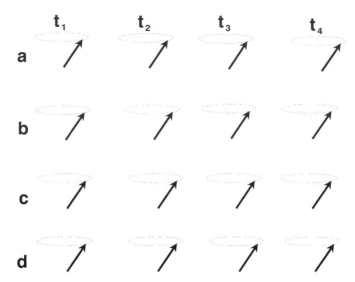

Figure 3–13A.   Four atoms (a, b, c, and d) precessing and viewed at 4 different times (t1, t2, t3, and t4). All atoms at all times are precessing together. At every time they are all in phase.

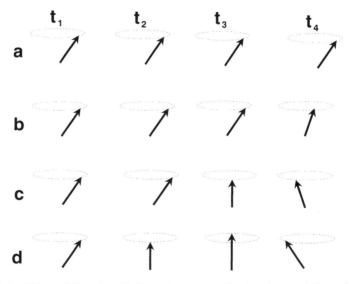

Figure 3–13B.   At time t1, all atoms are precessing in phase. At time t2, atom d is out of phase. At time t3, atoms c and d are out of phase with a and b. At time t4, all atoms are out of phase with one another.

rapidly than the longitudinal relaxation, so that the T2 value is much shorter than the T1 value. Typical T1 relaxation times for biological tissues range from 200 to 1,000 ms, whereas characteristic T2 relaxation times range from 50 to 150 ms. At higher applied magnetic fields, more atoms are aligned with the field and the T1 relaxation time is increased. T2 relaxation times are caused by local effects and are unaffected by field strengths.

In actual practice the T2 decay is faster than would be expected from the pure T2 value of the tissue being imaged. In addition to the actual T2 effect there are inhomogeneities in the local magnetic field around each nuclei which make the actual dephasing go faster. These field inhomogeneities are caused by variations in the applied magnetic field, changes in magnetic susceptibilities, chemical shifts, and changes caused by spins of nuclei moving in vascular tissues. The effective relaxation time for the actual process is called T2* (pronounced T-2 star).

During the relaxation process, the atoms emit rf energy of exactly the same energy that they had absorbed; these atomic magnets return to the equilibrium state that they were in before they absorbed the rf energy. This energy that is emitted by the atoms is responsible for generating the MR image (Chapter 4). The T1 relaxation process is primarily affected by the magnetic field of the overall environment, while the T2 relaxation is predominantly affected by the magnetic field in the local vicinity. The rf signal that is given off by the atoms returning to equilibrium is detected by an antenna and analyzed by computer techniques. For MR spectroscopy, a complex spectrum is obtained, while for MR imaging, the signal is translated into an image.

REFERENCES

1. Block F, Hansen WW, Packard ME. Nuclear induction. *Phys. Rev.* 1946; 69: 127.
2. Purcell EM, Torrey HC, Pound RV. Resonance absorption by nuclear magnetic moments in a solid. *Phys. Rev.* 1946; 69: 37.
3. Damadian R: Tumor detection by nuclear magnetic resonance. *Science.* 1971; 171: 1151.
4. Lauterbur P. Image formation by induced local interactions, examples employing nuclear magnetic resonance. *Nature.* 1973; 242: 190.

POINTS TO PONDER

....

- The nuclei of hydrogen atoms behave like magnets.

- The units of force of a magnetic field are gauss (G) and tesla (T), with 1 T equalling 10,000 G.

- The hydrogen nuclei are spinning around an axis.

- The spinning nuclei also precess, like a wobbly spinning top.

- When placed in a magnetic field, the hydrogen nuclei line up in the direction of the applied magnetic field and reach an equilibrium state.

- Electromagnetic energy, in the form of radiofrequency (rf) waves, is used to disturb the equilibrium of the aligned hydrogen atoms.

- Only specific rf energy, corresponding to the Larmor frequency, can be used to disturb the equilibrium. This rf energy is referred to as an rf pulse.

- After the rf pulse is stopped, the hydrogen nuclei will begin to re-attain the equilibrium state. A measure of the time to regain 63% of equilibrium is called the relaxation time.

- As the nuclei regain equilibrium, they release the rf energy that they had absorbed. This rf signal is called free induction decay.

- Regaining equilibrium occurs in two steps: T1, or longitudinal relaxation, which is dependent upon the overall magnetic field; and T2, or transverse relaxation, which is dependent upon the microscopic magnetic environment.

- T2* relaxation times take into account microscopic field inhomogeneities that causes T2 decay to occur more rapidly than expected.

CHAPTER FOUR

PRINCIPLES OF MAGNETIC RESONANCE IMAGING

The transition from understanding the principles of magnetic resonance to obtaining an image using MR is not a simple one. In 1973, nuclear magnetic resonance was first proposed as a potential imaging method for biological tissues. Dr. Paul Lauterbur, then working at Stony Brook, is credited with being the first to establish the complex method of obtaining images using the magnetic resonance properties of nuclei.[1] Since that time advances have come at a furious pace, with both hardware and software improvements continually being developed and new diagnostic uses being reported almost monthly in major journals.

In the previous chapter we saw that the nuclei of hydrogen atoms would align themselves parallel to an applied magnetic field. These nuclei could shift from the low energy state (aligned with the field) to the high energy state (aligned opposite to the field) if they acquired the proper energy, as specified by the Larmor equation. Eventually, these "excited" nuclei would return to their equilibrium state by giving off the energy that they had absorbed, dropping into the low-energy state again. It is this escaping energy that eventually permits an image to be created.

The signal obtained in the production of an MR image is determined by the total magnetic moment of all of the protons in each voxel. The magnetic moment can be most easily treated as a vector, so it is useful to review vectors and their properties before continuing further. A **vector** is a quantity that has both magnitude (or size) and direction. If we describe a car as traveling at 60 mph, we are only specifying magnitude (Figure 4–1A); if the car is traveling at 60 mph due west, we are describing a vector quantity (velocity) that has magnitude (60 mph) AND direction (due west) (Figure 4–1B). Similarly, magnetic moments are vector quantities and have magnitude and direction. A coordinate system is used to locate the position of a point. The direction associated with magnetic moments is given in terms of a normal three-dimensional coordinate system, with x, y, and z axes.

The usual x,y,z coordinate system is called the Cartesian coordinate system and is illustrated in Figure 4–2. It is named for René Descartes, French philosopher and mathematician, who lived from 1596 to 1649. His coordinate system was the unifying element between algebra and geometry. In this three-dimensional coordinate system, each axis is at a 90° angle to each of the other two. The center of the coordinate system can be pictured as the corner of a room: one axis runs from the corner along the line between the floor and one wall; another axis runs between the floor and the other wall; the third axis, the z axis, runs between

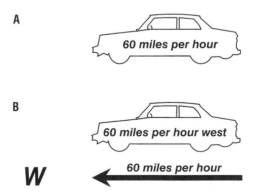

Figure 4–1.   (A) A car going 60 miles per hour cannot be considered a vector quantity: it has dimension (60 mph) but no direction is specified. (B) If we state that the car is traveling due west, we now have defined a vector quantity.

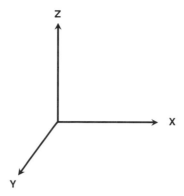

Figure 4–2. A normal three-dimensional Cartesian coordinate system has three axes: an *x* axis, a *y* axis, and a *z* axis. Each axis is at a 90° angle to the other two axes.

the two walls, up towards the ceiling. A vector can be represented by an arrow, which has both size (the length of the arrow) and direction (the way in which the arrow is pointing). In the coordinate system, this means that the size of the magnetic moment is represented by the length of the vector, and the direction of the field is the direction that the vector is pointing.

First let us examine the properties of a vector in a two-dimensional coordinate system, which has an *x* and a *y* axis (Figure 4–3A). A vector can be positioned in the coordinate system (Figure 4–3B). Every vector can be divided into its components that lie along the axis. The vector in Figure 4–3B has been divided into its *x* and *y* components in Figure 4–3C. The combination of these two vectors is exactly equal to the original vector. We can therefore either speak about the single vector of Figure 4–3B, or about its two components presented in Figure 4–3C, as either designation indicates the same quantity.

We can extend this process to three dimensions by considering the vector in Figure 4–4A. This vector has a component in each of the three axes, shown individually in Figures 4–4B–D, and all three components are illustrated together with the original vector in Figure 4–4E. The three components of the vector shown in Figure 4–4F are another, exactly equivalent way of indicating the information present in the single vector of Figure 4–4A.

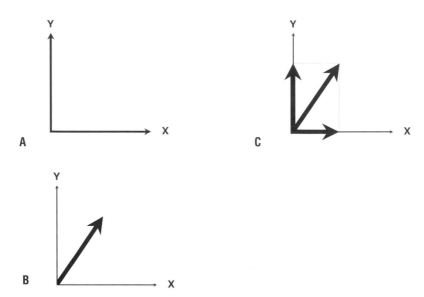

Figure 4–3.   (A) A two-dimensional Cartesian coordinate system has only two axes: an *x* axis and a *y* axis. (B) A vector has been placed in the coordinate system, extending from the origin (center). (C) The vector can be divided into individual components, one along each axis. The vector that lies along the *x* axis is referred to as the *x* component of the original vector; the vector that lies along the *y* axis is referred to as the *y* component of the original vector.

In the previous chapter we observed that the phenomenon of magnetic resonance occurs when atoms with magnetic moments that are aligned in a magnetic field are provided with the proper rf energy. These atomic magnets are spinning on their axes and are also precessing, or wobbling, as they spin (Figure 4–5).

During the production of an MR image, the receiver coil (acting as an antenna) picks up a signal in the *xy* plane. A moving magnetic field induces an electrical signal in a wire or an antenna. Since the atomic magnets are precessing, they are moving and thus induce a signal in the antenna. The frequency of the signal is identical to the Larmor frequency. The size, or magnitude, of the signal depends upon how much magnetization is present in the voxel being imaged.

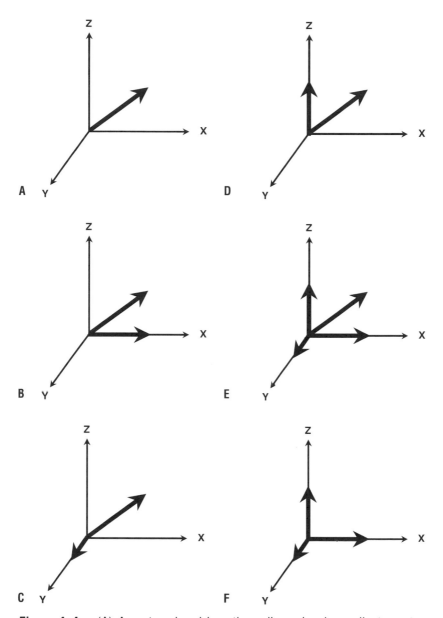

Figure 4–4.   (A) A vector placed in a three-dimensional coordinate system. (B) The *x* component of the vector. (C) The *y* component of the vector. (D) The *z* component of the vector. (E) The original vector, shown along with its components along each axis. (F) The original vector in A is equivalent to the three individual components pictured here.

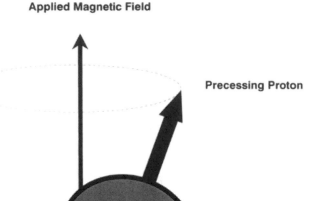

Figure 4–5.   In addition to spinning, the nuclear magnet precesses around the axis of the applied magnetic field.

The magnetization vector in the xy plane is designated as M_{xy}, and that along the z axis is M_z. Magnetization along the z axis does not add to the signal. In order to measure a signal in MR imaging, it is only the vector in the xy plane that provides information for the signal. Therefore, the larger the size of the M_{xy} vector, the larger the MR signal obtained. The xy plane is called the transverse plane, and so magnetization in this plane, M_{xy}, is referred to as **transverse magnetization**. The z axis is designated as the longitudinal direction; therefore magnetization along the z axis, M_z, is termed the **longitudinal magnetization**.

If we now consider the vector representing magnetic moments, we can use the same approach. Figure 4–6A illustrates the net magnetic vector (M) after a collection of atomic magnets have been knocked out of equilibrium by an rf pulse. This vector has three components, one along the z axis ($\mathbf{M_z}$), one along the x axis ($\mathbf{M_x}$), and one along the y axis ($\mathbf{M_y}$) (Figure 4–6B–E). These vectors can be rearranged to combine the x and y vectors into one vector ($\mathbf{M_{xy}}$), as shown in Figure 4–6F.

In order to increase the size of the transverse magnetization, an rf pulse is applied to "tip" the magnetic vector into the xy plane. This pulse is called an **excitation pulse**. In spin echo imaging, the pulse used most often is one in which the magnetic vector is tipped over by 90° (Figure 4–7). After a 90° flip, the longitudinal magnetization, $\mathbf{M_z}$, is equal to zero, with all of the initial magnetization converted into transverse magnetization, $\mathbf{M_{xy}}$. Once the pulse is turned off, the system begins to return to equilibrium, with the transverse magnetization decreasing and the longitudinal magnetization increasing. Although a 90° angle is used in spin echo imaging, any angle can be used in practice. In inversion recovery sequences, the initial pulse is a 180° rotation, and in gradient echo imaging, angles less than 90° are routinely used (Figure 4–8).

Let us consider a volume element that has been rotated through an angle of 90°. There are two different processes that occur as the system returns to equilibrium. The first process is called **longitudinal relaxation**, or **T1 relaxation**. (Relaxation is the term applied to a system returning to equilibrium.) Figure 4–9 depicts a series of vectors at different times. Before the 90° pulse is applied, all of the magnetization is along the z axis: there is no component in the xy plane. After the pulse is applied, the vector has been rotated into the xy plane so that all of the magnetization lies in the transverse plane; no longitudinal magnetization, $\mathbf{M_z}$, remains. As time progresses, $\mathbf{M_{xy}}$ decreases and $\mathbf{M_z}$ increases, until the system has fully recovered and all the magnetization has returned to lie along the z axis.

This process of $\mathbf{M_z}$ increasing, or recovering, as time increases after the rf pulse is shown in Figure 4–10. The increase in signal shown in this graph is called the **T1 recovery curve**. Materials with short T1 values, such as fat, will produce a higher signal in shorter times. If long enough periods of time are considered, signals from short T1 and long T1 materials will be equivalent. T1 relaxation values, therefore, will affect scans most

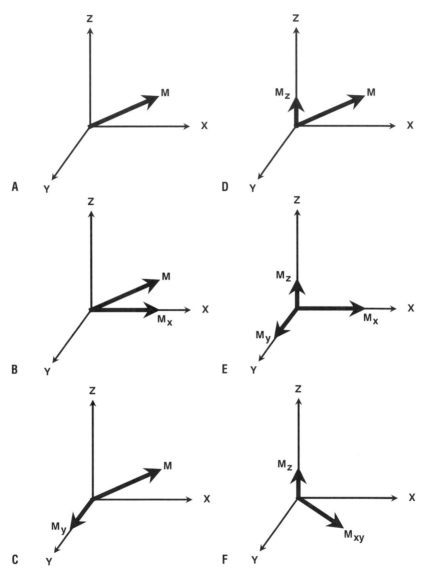

Figure 4–6.   (A) A magnetic vector, **M**, is placed in a coordinate system. (B) The component of the magnetic vector along the *x* axis can be represented by the vector **M**$_x$. (C) The component of the magnetic vector along the *y* axis can be represented by the vector **M**$_y$. (D) The component of the magnetic vector along the *z* axis can be represented by the vector **M**$_z$. (E) The original vector in A can be replaced by the three components **M**$_x$, **M**$_y$, and **M**$_z$. This combination is mathematically equivalent to the vector displayed in A. (F) Using a reverse process, the vectors **M**$_x$ and **M**$_y$ can be combined to the vector **M**$_{xy}$. The original vector in A can then be replaced by the combination of the vectors **M**$_z$ and **M**$_{xy}$.

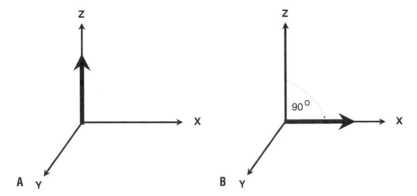

Figure 4–7.   (A) A magnetic vector along the z axis is referred to as the longitudinal magnetization. (B) After the proper rf pulse, the longitudinal magnetization can be flipped 90°. The vector in the xy plane is referred to as the transverse magnetization.

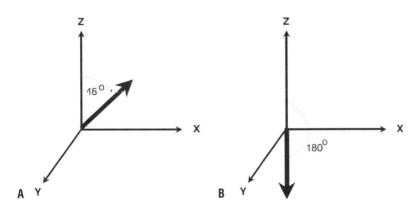

Figure 4–8.   (A) Gradient echo images use flip angles of less than 90°, as illustrated by the 45° flip in this example. (B) Both spin echo and inversion recovery sequences utilize 180° flip angles.

at relatively short times. T1 relaxation involves the nuclei giving up their energy to the surrounding environment. In a crystal, the environment is a lattice and the process is also called **spin-lattice relaxation**.

The second relaxation process that occurs involves changes in the transverse magnetization, $\mathbf{M}_{xy}$, and is called transverse relaxation or T2 relaxation. In order to understand T2 relaxation, we first want to discuss the concept of **phase**. When two or more

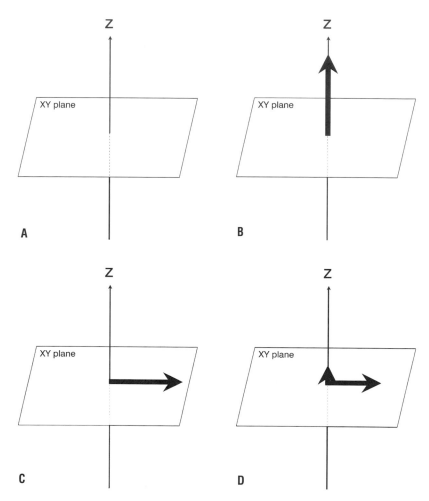

Figure 4–9. (A) The z axis runs perpendicular to the *xy* plane. Vectors along the z axis represent longitudinal magnetization; vectors in the *xy* plane represent transverse magnetization. (B) When placed in a magnetic field, the magnetic vector aligns along the z axis. (C) After a 90° rf pulse is applied, the magnetic vector is flipped into the *xy* plane. Longitudinal magnetization has been changed into transverse magnetization.

objects are **in phase**, they are traveling together; when they are **out of phase**, they are not traveling together. A squad of soldiers marching on a drill field is an example of objects in phase. Each soldier is standing erect and marching in the same direction as the rest of the squad, moving his right foot at the same time as

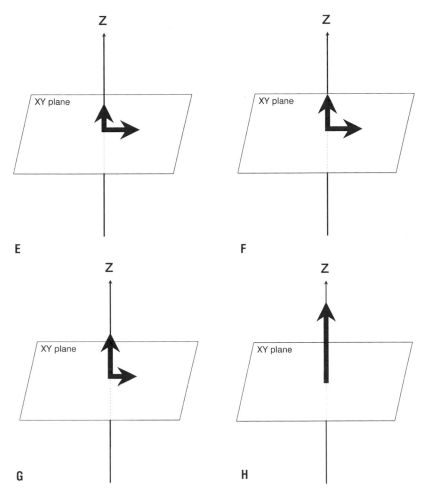

Figure 4–9 (*cont.*)   (D–G) As the system relaxes and returns to equilibrium, the amount of transverse magnetization decreases and the longitudinal magnetization increases. (H) Finally, the system has fully recovered and all of the magnetization again lies along the *z* axis.

every other soldier, and moving his left foot together with the rest. When the squad is dismissed, each soldier walks away at a different pace and in a different direction. The soldiers can now be said to be totally out of phase. An analogy closer to our precessing protons can be found if we consider several children

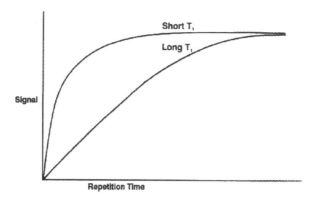

Figure 4–10.   T1 relaxation increases as time increases. Tissues with different T1 values behave differently, with those with shorter T1 values producing a higher signal in shorter times.

spinning tops. If they all spin their tops at the same time, at first they will all be spinning straight up. In this situation they are all doing the same thing and are in phase. As time goes by and some of them start to lose energy, they will start to wobble, or precess. They will all be wobbling, or precessing, at different rates and will start to get out of phase. The longer we wait, the more tops will begin to wobble; eventually each top will be pre-cessing at a different rate and they will be totally out of phase.

This same phenomenon occurs with our precessing mag-netic vectors. At equilibrium, before the rf pulse is applied, all the magnetic vectors are precessing together. At the instant that the 90° pulse is applied, they are all flipped into the *xy* plane but are still together in phase. After a few moments, some of the nuclei begin to precess at slightly different rates (or frequencies), and the system starts to go out of phase. As more and more nuclei precess differently, the system becomes more and more out of phase until all nuclei are precessing at different frequen-cies and the system is totally out of phase. This process is called **transverse relaxation,** or **T2 relaxation**. During T2 relaxation, all of the nuclei **dephase** their spins by transferring energy to neighboring atoms. This process is sometimes referred to as **spin-spin relaxation**. The decrease in signal obtained from T2 relaxation is shown in Figure 4–11. If the nuclei are in phase, their magnetic vectors in the *xy* plane are all pointing in the same direction and there is transverse magnetization. When they are totally out of phase, they are pointing in all different directions and cancel each other out, so there is no net magnetization in the *xy* plane (Figure 4–12). T2 values are much lower than T1 values, and the decay in T2 values is exponential. Tissues with short T2 relaxation times will give less signal than tissues with long T2 relaxation times, as shown on the graph in Figure 4–11.

After the rf pulse has flipped the magnetic moment into the *xy* plane, we will receive a signal in the antenna from each voxel in the sample being imaged. If all of the protons in the tissue emitted precisely the same rf frequency radiowaves, it would be impossible for the computer to determine where the protons were and to generate an image. In order to be able to obtain enough information to generate an image, spatial encoding information is added by altering the basic magnetic resonance unit. Magnetic field gradients are superimposed upon the static magnetic field.

A gradient is a rate of change. A magnetic field gradient implies that a slight change has been applied to the magnetic field, as illustrated along one dimension in Figure 4–13. At each point, A through F, the total magnetic field is slightly different,

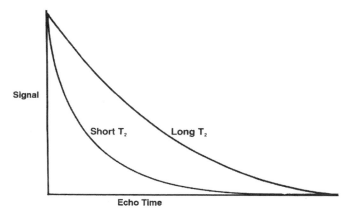

Figure 4–11.   T2 relaxation decreases as time increases. Tissues with different T2 values behave differently: those with short T2 values lose signal more rapidly than those with higher T2 values.

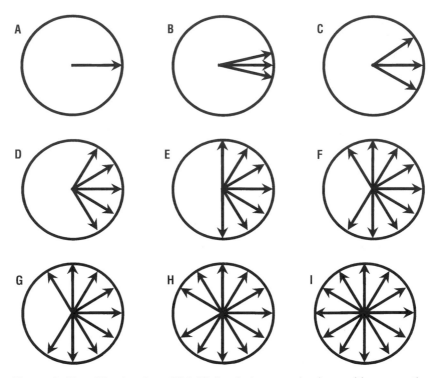

Figure 4–12. T2 relaxation. (A) Initially all atoms are in phase with one another. (B) After the cessation of the rf pulse, different atoms begin to precess at different rates, becoming increasingly out of phase with one another (C–H) until all atoms are totally out of phase (I).

being lowest at point A and highest at point F. Because of the Larmor equation, at each point, A through F, there will be a slightly different rf frequency that will cause resonance. Illustrative values are noted for each point above the diagram. Since atoms at each point will absorb a slightly different frequency, they will also emit these slightly different frequencies when returning to equilibrium. These frequencies can be analyzed by the computer, with each specific frequency assigned to a particular position. Using differences in frequency to determine the location of a particular position is referred to as **frequency encoding**. On MRI scans, the axis in which frequency encoding is utilized is referred to as the frequency encoding axis (usually, but not necessarily, the x axis as the image is viewed).

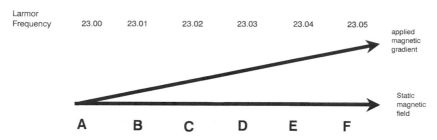

Figure 4–13. A magnetic gradient has been applied across the line from points A through F and is shown as its slope increases. Along each point the magnetic field is slightly different, so that the Larmor frequency at each point is slightly different and is indicated above the point.

Remaining with the one-dimensional analogy, suppose the signal analysis were to reveal the following:

Point	Frequency	Percentage
A	23.00	5%
B	23.01	18%
C	23.02	42%
D	23.03	20%
E	23.04	10%
F	23.05	5%

The computer would respond by making points A and F black, point E dark gray, points B and D, lighter gray and point C very bright. For a three-dimensional system, the mechanics are more complex, but the basic idea of how these gradients affect production of an image is the same.

In an actual MRI system, magnetic gradients are imposed in all three dimensions. One gradient is placed perpendicular to the plane of the anatomic section being imaged, and this is referred to as the **slice-selection gradient**. Since the static applied magnetic field is usually said to be applied in the z direction, the slice-selection gradient would be placed along the z axis for an axial section, along the y axis for a coronal section, and along the x axis for a sagittal section. The second gradient is the **frequency-encoding gradient**, which permits information to be obtained about the location of voxels in the x direction (for an axial section). The frequency-encoding gradient is applied twice during the imaging sequence, once at the beginning and once at the end of the imaging sequence. The third gradient, placed along the y axis, is referred to as the **phase-encoding gradient.**

In a column of voxels along a particular point on the x axis, all of the hydrogen nuclei will resonate at the same frequency, so a method must be used to distinguish among signals coming from the different positions along the y axis. This is accomplished by the use of a phase-encoding gradient. This magnetic gradient is applied early in the imaging sequence and has the effect of changing the precessional frequency of the nuclei in the different voxels. During the time that this gradient is applied, those nuclei at the higher fields will precess at a higher frequency than those at lower fields. After the gradient is stopped, all nuclei in the column of voxels will precess at the same frequency again; however, they will be out of phase with one another. Each voxel will therefore have a unique set of phase and frequency values, so that computer analysis can determine the strength of the signal emanating from each voxel in the slice. Figure 4–14 illustrates the effects of phase and frequency encoding on a 4-by-6 matrix. There are six gradient steps along the x axis and four gradient steps along the y axis. Frequency encoding is used along the x axis, so that each voxel has a different frequency. Notice that the frequencies in any column along the y axis are all the same. Phase encoding allows differentiation of the voxels along the y axis. No two voxels have the same phase and frequency. Each set is unique so that a computer analysis of the phase and frequency will determine exactly how much signal comes from each voxel and thus allow an image to be formed.

As noted in the previous chapter, a pulse of rf energy corresponding to the Larmor frequency will produce a magnetic resonance signal (FID). A single pulse will not provide enough information for imaging techniques, so this pulse must be repeated multiple times. The interval at which this pulse is repeated is appropriately called the **repetition time** and is abbreviated as **TR**. The repetition time is usually given in milliseconds (1 second = 1,000 ms). A TR of 3,000 ms (3 seconds) means that the rf pulse is repeated every 3 seconds. As we shall see, the time

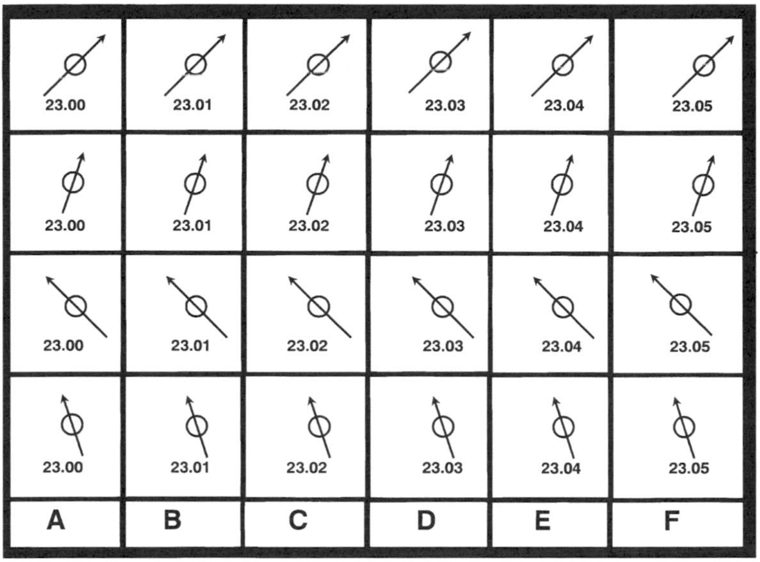

Figure 4–14. A 6-by-4 pixel matrix. A magnetic gradient is applied from left to right so that each column of pixels will resonate at the same frequency and pixels in the same row will resonate at a different frequency. A phase-encoding gradient is applied from top to bottom, so that in each row all pixels are in phase, and each pixel in each column is out of phase with the others. *No two pixels have the same combination of phase and frequency.*

between these pulses is not "wasted," but is put to good use. The rf pulse can be produced in order to flip the magnetization to any desired angle: for spin echo imaging, 90° and 180° pulses are the most useful. The repetition time determines how much longitudinal, or T1, relaxation occurs. The choice of TR will control the relative T1 contribution to the image. Another way of saying the same thing is that the TR controls the T1 weighting of the image.

The FID signal that is normally produced after an rf pulse induces magnetic resonance will not yield the information necessary to build an image. In order to obtain a signal capable of generating an image, the signal produced must be focused so that a large signal appears at a certain time. This focused signal is called an **echo**, and the amount of time it takes to appear after the rf pulse is applied is called the **echo time**, abbreviated **TE**. An echo is produced from the nuclei remaining in the transverse plane. In this plane, the precessing nuclei are dephasing—their precession occurs at different rates, some faster, some slower. At a given time, a **refocusing pulse**, usually 180°, is applied at half the echo time (TE/2). This refocusing pulse flips the entire system into essentially its mirror image. Those nuclei precessing at a faster rate still precess faster, but they are now going in the opposite direction and are now behind the slower precessing nuclei. This phenomenon effectively puts the slower precessing nuclei "into the lead," being chased by the faster nuclei. At the echo time, TE, all nuclei have reached the same point and the receiver coil detects a large signal, which is referred to as an echo.

The 180° refocusing pulse can be thought of in terms of an automobile race. Suppose that we have three cars in the race; car A can travel 30 miles per hour, which is equivalent to 44 feet per second; car B can travel at 45 miles per hour, or 66 feet per second; car C can travel at 60 miles per hour, or 88 feet per second. Obviously as time progresses all three cars will be at different points, with car C in the lead. In this race, however, we have an added feature: at some given time we send out a signal that all cars have to turn around immediately and head back to the starting line. (This is equivalent to our refocusing pulse). As an example, let us say that we allow the cars to race for 100 seconds before giving the signal to turn around. Car A will have traveled 4,400 feet from the starting line; car B will have traveled 6,600 feet; car C will have traveled 8,800 feet. Now they instantly turn around and head back to the starting line. Car A is in the lead, has only 4,400 feet to go, and will need 100 seconds to reach the starting line. Car B is in second place, 6,600 feet away, and will also need 100 seconds to reach the starting line. Car C now finds itself in last place, 8,800 feet away, and will also reach the starting line in 100 seconds. By turning all of the cars around (using our refocusing pulse), they all arrive at the starting line together. This is equivalent to all of our nuclei precessing out of phase, then being refocused so that they produce a strong signal—and all arriving back in phase together at the echo time, TE. The choice of TE will determine the relative contribution of transverse relaxation, or T2 relaxation, to the overall signal. The choice of TE, therefore, determines the amount of T2 weighting of the image.

POINTS TO PONDER

- Magnetic moments can be treated as a vector.

- Vectors have both magnitude (size) and direction.

- Any vector can be broken down into its components along each axis or a coordinate system.

- The magnetic moment along the z axis is called the longitudinal magnetization and is represented by the symbol $\mathbf{M}_z$.

- The magnetic moment in the xy plane is called the transverse magnetization and is represented by the symbol $\mathbf{M}_{xy}$.

- Only transverse magnetization, $\mathbf{M}_{xy}$, will produce a signal for an MR image.

- The process of obtaining an image is started by applying an rf pulse of the proper frequency to "tip" or "flip" the longitudinal magnetization off the z axis so that there will be some component in the xy plane.

- For spin echo imaging, the flip angle is 90°.

- Relaxation is a term used to describe a system returning to equilibrium.

- Longitudinal, or T1, relaxation is the gradual decrease in the transverse magnetization, $\mathbf{M}_{xy}$, and corresponding increase in longitudinal magnetization, $\mathbf{M}_z$.

- Objects are in phase when they are moving together, and out of phase when they are not.

- Transverse, or T2, relaxation is the gradual dephasing of spins and loss of transverse magnetization.

- T1 relaxation results from the loss of energy by the nuclei to the environment.

- T2 relaxation results from the loss of energy due to the interaction of nuclei with their neighboring nuclei.

POINTS TO PONDER *(continued)*

- To generate an image, a magnetic gradient is applied in the x dimension, causing each voxel to have a slightly different magnetic field, therefore resonating at a slightly different rf frequency.

- A phase-encoding gradient is applied in the y dimension to permit each voxel to have a unique set of frequency and phase components, allowing an image to be formed.

- The time between rf pulses is called the repetition time, or TR.

- The repetition time controls the relative T1 weighting of images.

- A refocusing pulse is applied to rephase the nuclei and produce a large signal. The refocusing pulse is applied at a time TE/2, and the signal is generated at time TE, the echo time.

- The echo time, TE, controls the relative T2 weighting of images.

REFERENCES

1. Lauterbur P. Image formation by induced local interactions, examples employing nuclear magnetic resonance. *Nature*. 1973; 242: 190.

COMPONENTS OF MAGNETIC RESONANCE IMAGING SYSTEMS

Magnetic resonance imaging systems are complex combinations of instrumentation, which continue to become more sophisticated as advances in imaging continue. MRI systems are usually classified as low-field (below 0.2 T), mid-field (between 0.2 T and 0.6 T), and high-field (1.0 T and above). As diagrammed in Figure 5–1, the various components, computers, and electronics, have a complex interrelationship, combined in such a manner as to provide homogeneous magnetic fields and to produce the highest-quality images possible.

The fundamental starting point in the production of a magnetic resonance imaging system is the magnet. As mentioned previously, there are essentially three different types of magnets available: permanent magnets, electromagnets (also called resistive magnets), and superconducting magnets. Each type of magnet can be used to manufacture an MRI system, and each system has advantages and disadvantages. Since the majority of MRI units in operation are superconducting systems, which are necessary for field strengths of 0.5 T and higher, most of the discussion will be centered on these units.

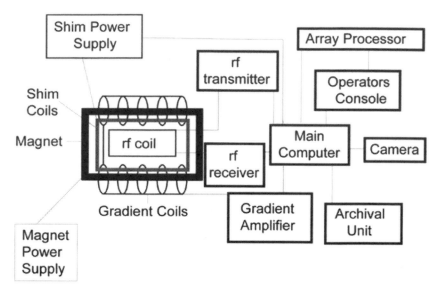

Figure 5–1. Schematic diagram of an MR imaging system illustrating the interrelationships among the various components necessary to obtain an image.

Imaging systems using permanent magnets were the first to be produced, historically. They are easier to produce than the other types of systems, and they are the least expensive to purchase. In order to obtain magnetic fields high enough to produce an image, the magnet must be quite large; these units become extremely heavy, weighing in excess of 100 tons. Finding a proper site for a permanent MR unit becomes a problem because of the excessive weight, and most of these systems must be placed on solid ground. Field strengths are relatively low, ranging up to 0.2 T, so that the signal-to-noise (SNR) ratio is low. This low field strength either will produce images of diminished resolution or will significantly increase scanning time to compensate for the relatively low SNR. Permanent magnets offer several key advantages: they have low operational costs; no electric power is necessary; and the fringe field, the field around the magnet, drops off sharply so that no shielding is necessary.

Resistive systems use an electromagnet in order to generate the necessary magnetic field. These are also relatively low-field systems, producing imaging fields up to approximately 0.35 T. These units are considerably less expensive than superconducting systems; however, since an electrical current is needed continuously to provide the magnetic field, operating costs are high. With the continuous current, there is a significant heating effect, so the unit must be equipped with a cooling system, usually circulating water. The resistive system is lighter than a permanent system, but it does have an appreciable fringe field. Permanent and resistive systems can be combined to produce hybrid magnetic imaging systems, which keep a permanent magnetic core with wires coiled around it (as in a resistive system). The field strength is only slightly higher than obtained with a resistive system (0.35 T), but it requires less electrical power, so that operating costs are lower. Once thought to be the best compromise between image quality and functional cost, hybrid systems are no longer as popular as they once were.

Superconducting MRI systems are currently the most popular type of unit utilized for patient studies. The main advantage of superconducting magnets is that they provide the highest field strengths available for imaging, up to 1.5 T. This high field strength produces the highest intrinsic SNR as well as the highest resolution images per unit imaging time. These systems are the most complex (Figure 5–2) and also the most expensive. The metallic coils must be cooled to liquid helium temperatures, so the magnet must be encased in a housing containing liquid helium. In order to minimize the evaporation of the liquid helium, it in turn is encased in a jacket containing liquid nitrogen, or, in the more recent systems, refrigeration coils. Both jackets containing the liquid helium and liquid nitrogen are surrounded by vacuum jackets in order to minimize the entry of heat, which would boil off the low-temperature liquids.

In order to generate the magnetic field, a small amount of electric current must be applied when the system is first made operational. No further electrical current is necessary, as long as the temperature is kept below the critical temperature of the metal. Although no significant power is necessary, cryogen (liquid helium and liquid nitrogen) costs can be high, especially in older units. Units currently being manufactured require cryogen fills only four to six times a year, but older systems require filling every

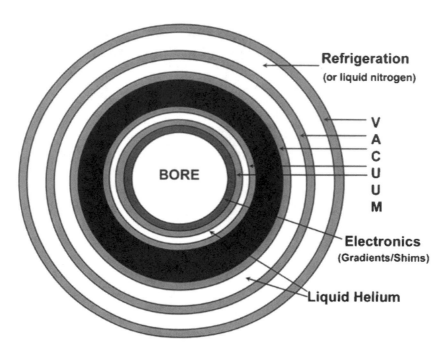

Figure 5–2. Cross-sectional view through a superconducting MRI unit. The patient is placed within the bore. The bore is lined with gradient coils and body rf transmit/receive coils that are cosmetically covered (not shown). Liquid helium surrounds the magnet to cool the metal to superconducting temperatures. The liquid helium, in turn, is surrounded by a jacket of either liquid nitrogen, or refrigeration coils, to minimize the amount of heat that might enter, thus minimizing the amount of helium from boiling off. Each layer is surrounded by vacuum layers to further prevent cryogen loss from heating.

two to four weeks. In newer systems, highly efficient refrigeration systems have replaced the liquid nitrogen as a method of preventing heat loss of liquid helium by evaporation. This is less costly and more efficient than continual filling with liquid nitrogen.

In any type of system, the most important requirement is that the magnetic field produced within the magnet's bore be as uniform as possible. The size of the bore affects the system's ability to maintain a homogeneous field: the larger the bore size, the more difficult it is to maintain a uniform magnetic field. This difficulty increases with increasing magnetic fields and is the reason why high-field-strength magnets have smaller bores than low-field-strength magnets. The so-called open magnets are able to maintain homogeneous magnetic fields with large openings for the patient because they are utilizing low field strengths. These large openings produce a much less "closed-in" feeling for the patient. There is, however, a trade-off, since at the low field strength the signal-to-noise ratio is much lower, so that the inherent resolution of the images obtained will also be lower.

A new type of system being developed, the interventional magnet, is an MRI unit that will permit radiologists or surgeons to perform interventional or therapeutic procedures while the patient is in the magnet. Figure 5–3 shows a prototype of an interventional magnet. There is an "open" space within the normal bore, allowing medical personnel to perform procedures and immediately check the effect on the patient with an MRI scan. This system has the potential to precisely treat lesions that could not be observed by CT scanning, and to immediately observe the effect of treatment and interventional procedures.

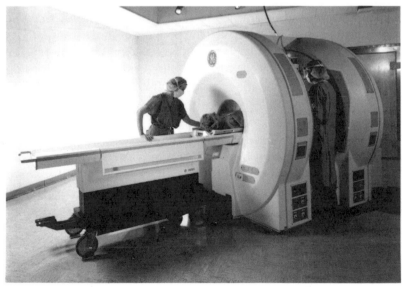

Figure 5–3. An interventional magnet. Notice the "open" area that allows nonmagnetic equipment to be utilized, precisely localized, and observed by MRI scanning immediately before and after MRI scans. (Courtesy of General Electric Medical Systems, Inc., Waukeshau, WI)

SHIELDING

Two completely different types of shielding are involved with MR imaging systems: **magnetic shielding,** used to contain the peripheral magnetic field around the magnet, and **rf shielding,** used to keep stray rf radiation out of the imaging room. Magnetic shielding is used to contain the fringe field around the magnet. Although there is no requirement, FDA guidelines recommend that areas over 5 G be restricted areas. The fringe field for 1.5 T systems can extend for considerable distances. Since space is usually a valuable commodity, most systems use some type of shielding to minimize the distance of the 5 G zone (Figures 5–4, 5–5, and 5–6).

Two different approaches have been employed to decrease the fringe field: either the magnet can be placed within a room that has steel shielding within the walls (essentially placing it within a steel box), or the shielding can be placed directly on the magnet. Shielding the room by lining the walls with iron is an effective method of containing the field, but it has significant drawbacks. The smaller the room, the thicker is the shielding that is required. Not only can this be expensive, but the shielding is quite heavy. Together with the weight of the magnet, it can introduce structural support problems. Any asymmetry in the positioning of the shielding can cause homogeneity problems within the bore of the magnet, as well.

There are two different techniques for placing the shielding directly on the magnet: active shielding and passive shielding. **Passive shielding** involves placing iron slabs directly on the magnet. It is effective but must be arranged very carefully in order to maintain a homogeneous magnetic field within the center of the bore. **Active shielding** uses coils of wire carrying electric currents—effectively small electromagnets—to counteract and reduce the peripheral fringe field. Figure 5–6 illustrates the magnetic lines of force for a passively shielded magnet.

The second type of shielding required around the magnet is rf shielding. Even a small amount of stray signal entering the magnet room can produce significant interference if it is within the proper frequency range. Since the Larmor frequencies for MR imaging systems lie in the upper FM and lower television

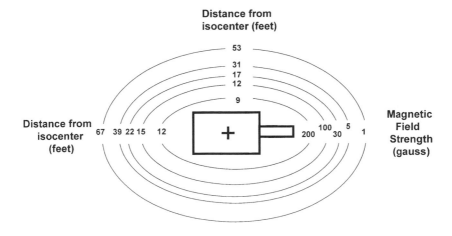

A   **1.5 Tesla Unshielded Magnet**

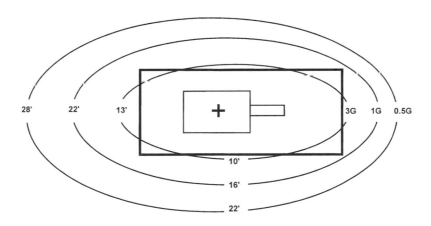

B   **1.5 Tesla Unshielded Magnet inside shielded room**

Figure 5–4. (A) Magnetic field strengths (in gauss) at different distances (in feet) from a nonshielded 1.5 T magnet. Actual lines are not as symmetric as shown, having a more irregular contour due to the size and shape of the magnet and the presence of external metal in beams, structural supports, and so on. (B) A similar diagram for a 1.5 T MRI system in a shielded room. The field strengths at comparable distances to that in A can be seen to be much less. The 5 G zone is kept within the confines of the room, less than 10 feet from the isocenter of the magnet, compared to 39 feet for the same magnet in open space.

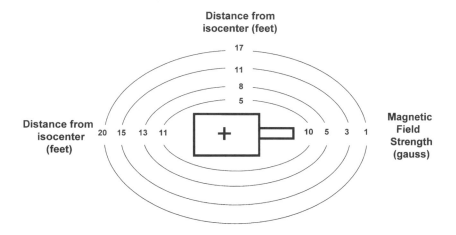

0.5 Tesla Magnet

Figure 5–5.   Compared to Figure 5–4, the magnetic field strength (in gauss) at different distances from a shielded 0.5 T magnet demonstrates a significant decrease in the distance of the fringe field, with the 5 G zone limited to 13 feet along the long axis of the magnet.

broadcast range, the magnet room must be completely insulated from interference from radio waves generated outside of the system. The magnet room is completely enclosed by copper shielding. Care must be taken that the room is completely sealed, with no rf leaks when the entry door is closed. Joints must be welded or lapped and bolted. During construction, extreme caution must be exercised not to accidentally ground the shielding and inadvertently turn it into an antenna.

All wires and cables are routed to a special box in the room, which is called a penetration panel. A penetration panel is set up so that all computer cables and electrical lines entering or leaving the room do not disrupt the seal. Electrical lines entering the enclosure must be adequately filtered. Fluorescent lighting within the scanning room can flicker if dimmed or defective and may produce rf radiation, which can interfere with the images.

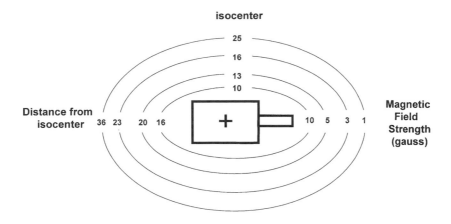

isocenter

Distance from isocenter   36   23   20   16

Magnetic Field Strength (gauss)

1.5 Tesla Passively Shielded Magnet

Figure 5–6.   When compared to Figure 5–4, the passively shielded 1.5 T magnet can be seen to contain the magnet field much more effectively, with the 5 G zone down to 20 feet from 39 feet.

SHIMS

In order to provide optimum imaging, the magnetic field must be homogeneous, within 10 ppm. The abbreviation **ppm** stands for "parts per million" and is a measure of how uniform the magnetic field is. In a 1 T field, for example, which equals 10,000 G, a homogeneity of 10 ppm would mean that the magnetic field does not vary from point to point by more than 0.1 G, or 0.000001 T. (For spectroscopy even greater homogeneity is required, and fields must be within 1 ppm.) A change in the magnetic field by a factor of only 3 ppm will shift the position of a signal by one pixel. This in turn will cause the appearance of an artificial structure in the image, referred to as an **artifact** (Chapter 10). In order to obtain true images, the magnetic field must be as homogeneous as possible.

The homogeneity of the magnetic field demands that the coils of either resistive or superconducting magnets be uniformly wound and equally spaced. Even a very small irregularity may cause an unacceptable variation in the field strength and would produce image distortions, blurring, or areas of absent signal. Large metallic objects in the area, such as elevator shafts, construction beams, electrical equipment, and so forth can also affect the homogeneity of the field within the bore of the magnet. Adjusting the homogeneity of the magnetic field to within acceptable levels is referred to as *shimming* the magnet.

One method used on permanent magnets, and to make minor corrections on resistive and superconductive systems, is to place small pieces of magnetic material within the bore of the magnet to correct variations. Although this appears to be a crude type of correction, experienced personnel are able to employ this method successfully. Resistive and superconducting units use shim coils, which are isolated additional loops of wire within the magnet. The shim power supply produces small amounts of current, which are passed through these coils and which will adjust the inhomogeneities in the magnetic field.

There are two types of shim coils: **resistive shims**, which are analogous to electromagnetic coils and require small amounts of current running through them constantly; and **superconducting shims**, which are small superconducting coils, which receive an electrical current only when the system is started up. Resistive shims are used in both resistive and superconducting systems, while superconducting shims are used only in superconducting systems. A single resistive shim power supply will typically control many independent coils, and only one of these electrical channels will fail at a given time, making detection difficult. These problems will usually result in a geometric distortion of the images (see Chapter 10).

GRADIENTS

In order to apply the magnetic gradients described in the previous chapter, gradient coils must be placed within the magnet. It is these gradient coils that produce the knocking noise that has become associated with MR imaging. The gradient coils are activated by pulsing electricity through them. They are encased in rigid plastic. The electrical pulses produce a very strong force, which causes the gradients to move. Even though they are embedded in a plastic cylinder, the force is strong enough to cause them to move and "bang" against the plastic that holds them. This produces the loud knocking noise.

Once the overall magnetic field of the imaging system has been properly established, the gradient coils are used to produce small, linear changes in the magnetic field within the bore so that images can be obtained. These coils are used only during imaging and require large amounts of electrical power. They must be turned off and on hundreds and sometimes thousands of times for each image produced. They change the magnetic field of each pixel within the bore of the magnet by very small amounts, usually less than 1 G per cm. Since three magnetic gradients are necessary, one each along the x, y, and z axes, three gradient coils are used (Figure 5–7). As previously mentioned, these gradients are used to permit slice selection and phase and frequency encoding.

The quality of the magnetic gradient coils is important in determining the eventual imaging parameters available to the operator. The gradient coils make changes in the magnetic field over certain distances by allowing small electrical currents to flow within the coils. Gradient amplifiers, one at each end of the

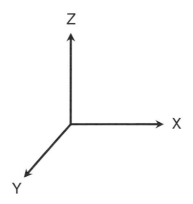

Figure 5–7.   A three-dimensional coordinate system is used, with the axes mutually perpendicular. The z direction is arbitrarily chosen as the direction of the primary magnetic field, and the x and y directions are in the imaging plane.

gradient coil, produce the electrical current needed. By proper adjustment of the gradient amplifiers, the changes in the magnetic field in any direction, called the **slope** of the magnetic field gradient, can be made smaller or larger. The slope of the magnetic field gradients becomes the limiting factor in determining the minimum slice thickness and the minimum field of view that can be obtained by the system. Very steep gradient slopes allow the unit to produce thin slices and small fields of view. These in turn produce images of higher resolution. Obtaining steeply sloped gradients and maintaining acceptable homogeneity of the magnetic field is a difficult engineering problem.

Designing stable gradient coils can be a difficult task, since gradient instability or nonuniformity will produce artifacts within the image. Gradient coils are powered by gradient amplifiers, one on the high end and one on the low end of the gradient coil. Magnetic gradients must be developed very rapidly during imaging, but too quick a change in magnetic field can induce small currents within the magnet called eddy currents. These eddy currents can cause inhomogeneity effects within the system; they are thus a source of image artifacts and must be minimized for proper image production. Defective, overheated, or unstable gradient amplifiers will produce a wide variety of image artifacts, most commonly involving blurring, ghosting, banding, or truncation in the phase-encoding direction. One method of minimizing eddy currents is in the use of shielded gradient coils. These consist of a pair of an inner and an outer coil, in which the inner coil produces the gradient changes necessary to the production of the image and the outer coil nullifies the effect of the gradient coil on other areas of the magnet.

RF COILS

The radiofrequency coils are an integral part of the imaging system, being used to transmit and receive the rf signal during the scan. The transmitting and receiving coils can be separate coils, or they can be a single, dual-purpose unit. Body coils, head coils, and surface coils are examples of rf coils. The rf pulse is produced by a frequency synthesizer and transmitted by the rf transmitter coil, acting in effect as a broadcast antenna. The transmitter is designed so that the rf pulse transmission will be homogeneous, and of proper pulse shape and intensity. Radiofrequency-associated problems, usually a lack of a signal, are more often due to the rf amplifiers than to the transmitter coil.

Once the MRI signal is produced, it is picked up by the receiving rf coil (acting as an antenna), and then sent through a pre-amplifier, a signal amplifier, and finally an analog-to-digital converter (ADC). This ADC changes the signal from an analog to a digital format so that it can be transmitted to the computer for processing into the MR image.

The body coil is an rf coil that is located within the housing of the magnet and is used to both transmit and receive. All other rf coils, such as the head coil, are placed within the bore of the magnet when they are to be used. Surface coils (also referred to local coils) are specially designed coils that are used to image specific areas of the body (lumbar spine, knee, temporomandibular joints, etc.) (Figure 5–8). These coils are shaped to fit as close to the area of interest as possible (to get the maximum possible signal), and they offer extremely high resolution and increased SNR, producing high-quality images of small anatomic structures (Figure 5–9). Surface coils can operate as transmitter coils, as receiver coils, or as combined transmit/receive coils.

Phased-array coils attempt to eliminate the compromise between field of view (FOV) and resolution associated with obtaining images. Surface coils will increase resolution by increasing the SNR, but at a cost of a decreased FOV, while body coils will image large FOVs, but at a decreased SNR or lower resolution. Ideally, the radiologist would prefer high resolution with large FOV images so that the high resolution obtained by surface coils on small body parts could be available for all parts of the body. Phased-array coils attempt to provide an answer to this problem. Multiple surface coils are arranged in a particular anatomic configuration to conform to the part of the body being imaged. For the abdomen or pelvis, these coils can be arranged around the body, while for the entire spine they can be grouped in a straight line. Each coil acts as an individual receiver, collecting data simultaneously but independently. Special software combines the data received from each coil and integrates it into a series of images covering a large area, having increased SNR and increased high resolution.

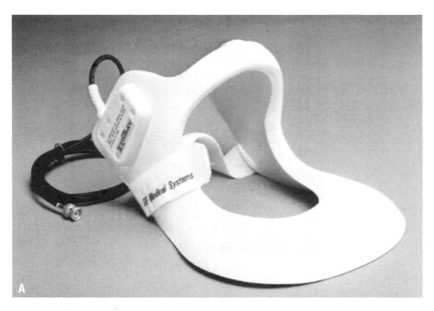

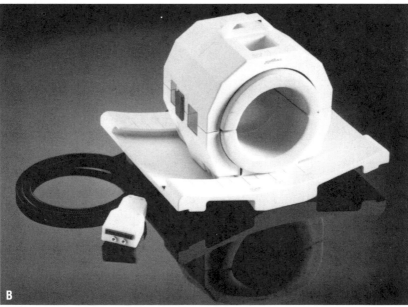

Figure 5–8. Several different types of surface coils, designed so that they will be as close to the area of interest as possible. (A) Anterior neck coil, a partial-volume coil that lies on top of the neck and sternum and does not completely surround the area of investigation. (B) Knee coil, a full-volume coil, which completely encases the knee.

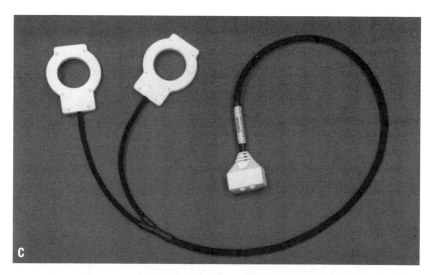

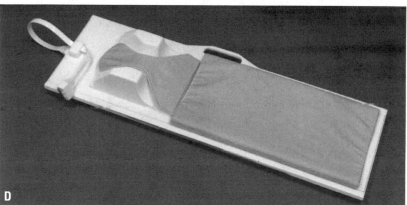

Figure 5–8. *(cont.)*   (C) Bilateral flat 3-in. coils used for imaging both orbits or both temporomandibular joints simultaneously. (D) Phased-array total-spine coil permitting the entire spine to be imaged with submillimeter resolution. (Courtesy of Medrad, Inc., Pittsburgh, PA)

Quadrature coils are rf coils designed to significantly improve SNR while decreasing the power necessary to produce superior images. These coils act as if they were two separate coils, arranged at a 90° angle relative to one another. This has the effect of producing a rotating rf field rather than a field aligned along a single axis. The rotating rf field interacts much more productively with tissues, increasing signal-to-noise and requiring much less rf power.

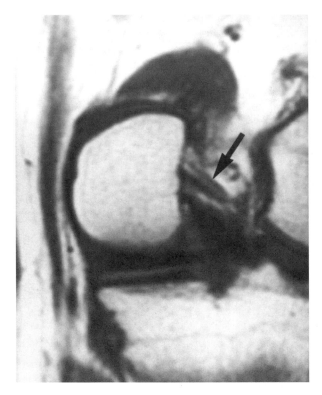

Figure 5–9. High-resolution surface coil image: coronal view through the posterior aspect of the knee, demonstrating small structures such as the ligament of Wrisberg (arrow), which is approximately 1 mm thick.

Radiofrequency artifacts can be observed as discrete lines or streaks on the image, if there is a leak in the rf shielding; as decreased signal and increased noise, if the amplifier is not operating properly; or as inhomogeneities or contrast abnormalities, if the rf tuning is faulty (Figure 5–10).

COMPUTER SYSTEM

The computer system is an integral part of the entire MRI unit, although most of the hardware is usually housed in a separate air-conditioned room. The system consists of multi-

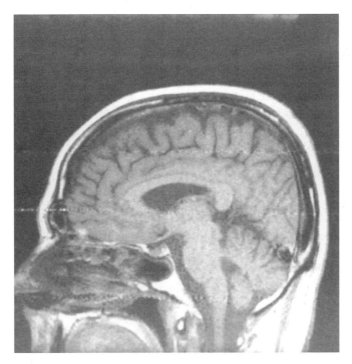

Figure 5–10. Linear streak artifacts are observed through the image obtained in a room in which the rf shielding was faulty.

ple components, including drivers for the gradient and rf systems; hardware and software for reconstruction and display; archival equipment; and the operating console. The most obvious—and most often used—part of the computer system to the patient and operator is the operator's console. The entire process of starting the system, scanning a patient, producing images, filming, and archiving can be controlled from here. The operator's console is dependent upon the array processor, which is required for rapid image processing. Using advanced mathematical techniques, such as Fourier transforms, the digitized FID signal for each pixel is converted into an appropriate shade of gray and displayed on the monitor.

POINTS TO PONDER

- MR imaging systems are classified as high-field (greater than 1.0 T), mid-field (between 0.2 T and 0.6 T), and low-field (below 0.2 T).

- MR images can be obtained using permanent, resistive, hybrid, or superconducting systems.

- Permanent magnets are relatively inexpensive with low operational costs, but they are heavy, have siting problems, and produce low magnetic fields.

- Resistive magnets are electromagnets, which produce higher magnetic fields than permanent systems but have high operating costs.

- Superconducting magnets produce very high magnetic fields and high SNR, need liquid helium to produce the temperatures necessary for superconductivity, and are the most expensive currently available.

- Fringe fields can be minimized either by magnetically shielding the magnet room or by applying shielding directly to the magnet.

- Passive shielding applies solid shielding directly to the magnet.

- Active shielding utilizes coils of current as small electromagnets to reduce the fringe field.

- Magnetic field inhomogeneity is corrected by using shims.

- Gradient coils are used to produce magnetic gradients separately in the x, y and z directions.

- Radiofrequency coils will act to transmit and receive rf signals.

- Surface coils are designed to produce high-resolution images of restricted areas of the body.

- Surface coils must be placed as close to the region of interest as possible.

- Phased array coils are a series of surface coils arranged to permit imaging of large areas of the body with high resolution.

POINTS TO PONDER *(continued)*

- Quadrature coils increase SNR and decrease power requirements by acting as two separate coils oriented at 90°, producing a rotating rf field.

- An array processor is added to the system for rapid image reconstruction.

6

IMAGING SEQUENCES

When beginning an imaging procedure, in addition to the part of the body to be imaged and the imaging planes desired, the type of pulse sequences to be used must be determined. The pulse sequence can be defined as the combination and timing of rf pulses used for the production of an image. In practical terms, these are the types of rf pulse (30°, 90°, 180°, etc.) used in the sequence, the amount of time in between these pulses, and the length of time until the sequence is repeated (which is TR, or the repetition time). The spin-echo sequence is the most commonly used pulse sequence. Figure 6–1 is a schematic diagram of the pulses used in obtaining a spin-echo image.

The MR appearance of the various types of tissues will be controlled by the T1 and T2 values, the proton density (or concentration of mobile hydrogen atoms in the tissue), and the presence of flow or diffusion. By the proper selection of pulse sequences, these different factors can be made to accentuate their contribution to the image to different degrees, permitting both anatomy and pathology to be highlighted in different images. In spin-echo imaging, for example, choosing low values of TE and TR will make the image very dependent upon the T1 values of the tissues (Figure 6–2A); this type of image is called a

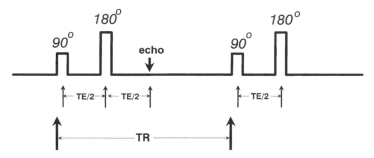

Figure 6–1.   To obtain a spin-echo image, a 90° rf pulse is followed by a rephasing pulse of 180°. The thick arrows indicate the beginning of the rf pulse. The time between the rf pulses (thick arrows) is the repetition time. The time between the center of the 90° pulse and the 180° pulse (thin arrows) represents half of the echo time, TE.

T1-weighted image. T1-weighted images have very high resolution, high signal-to-noise ratios (SNRs), and define the anatomy very well. They do not, in general, have a high degree of contrast between tissues. By choosing high values of TE and TR (making the scanning time much longer), the T2 values of the tissues make a larger contribution to the image quality; images so produced are called T2-weighted images (Figure 6–2C). T2-weighted images do not have as high a resolution as do T1-weighted images, but contrast between tissues is very high. It is in these T2-weighted images that pathology is most often identified. If intermediate values of TR and TE are chosen in spin-echo imaging from the equations that govern image intensity, the density of protons in the tissue is the most important factor in determining the quality of the image; images so produced are called proton-density images (Figure 6–2B).

Mathematically, signal intensity can be expressed in the following terms:

Signal intensity = A [N_0][1 – exp(–TR/T1)][exp(–TE/T2)]

where A is a proportionality constant, N_0 is the density of protons, and T1, T2, TR, and TE have their usual significance. If TE and TR are short, the last term approaches 1, the middle term becomes large, and the T1 value is most instrumental in determining the signal intensity; if TE and TR are long, the middle term approaches 1, the last term is large, and the T2 value determines signal intensity; in an intermediate situation, neither of the last two terms is large and the density of protons is significant in determining signal intensity.

A **pulse sequence** is the way in which combinations of rf pulses of various kinds can be used. The most common types of rf pulses are the 90° pulse and the 180° pulse, which cause the precessing nuclei to tip 90° and 180°, respectively, from the z axis. The flip angle can technically be of any value, and angles of 20°, 30°, and 60° are commonly used in gradient-echo and fast-scanning techniques. These different flip angles can be obtained by varying the strength of the rf pulse and the length of time that it is applied. In order to provide higher resolution, thinner sections, and fewer artifacts, in general shorter pulse times are preferred.

Spin-echo imaging is the most common type of MR imaging performed. Figure 6–1 shows the pulse sequence as a 90° pulse followed by a 180° pulse. This sequence is repeated over and over again. The time between repeated pulses is the repetition time, TR. The time between the mid-point of the 90° pulse and the refocusing pulse (180°) is equal to half of the echo time, TE. In Figure 6–1, the large arrows indicate when a new rf pulse is introduced. TR is shown as the time between the large arrows, and the time between the two pulses, TE/2, is the time between the small arrows. If the repetition time is long enough, several refocusing pulses can be employed before the rf is applied again (Figure 6–3). This pulse sequence will produce several images at different TE values. Each of these images is called a different echo. The longer the TE value, the more T2-weighted the image becomes (Figure 6–4). These echoes can be symmetric (e.g., 30 ms, 60 ms, 90 ms, 120 ms) or asymmetric echoes (e.g., 30 ms, 90 ms).

Timing diagrams are commonly seen when describing different pulse sequences. Although these diagrams may seem very difficult to interpret at first glance, they are simply a

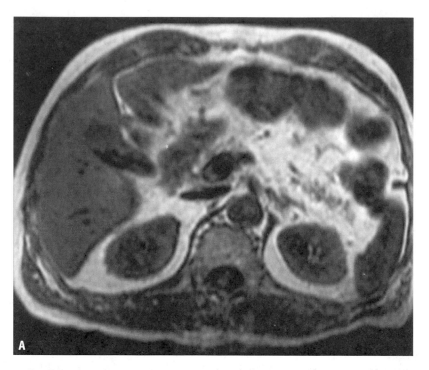

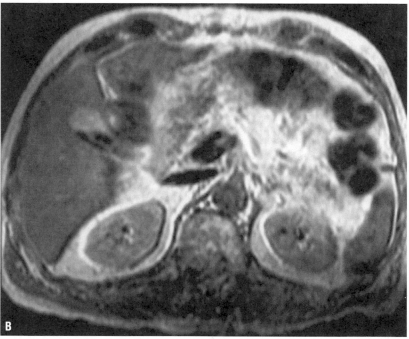

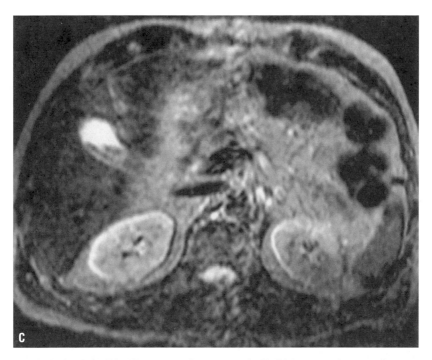

Figure 6–2. (A) T1, (B) proton density, and (C) T2 images through the liver illustrate the difference in signal intensity from the different structures as their T1 and T2 weighting changes.

method of indicating where the different rf pulses and gradients are placed in order to obtain the desired pulse sequence. Figure 6–5 shows five different linear graphs. The first (RF) indicates the timing of the rf pulses—in this case a normal spin-echo image. The second line (SIG) indicates where (at what time) the signal for the image appears. The peak of the signal is a time TE after the 90° rf pulse. The three bottom lines indicate what happens to the magnetic gradients along each of the three axes: G_x, the x-gradient, is a frequency-encoding gradient; G_y, the y-gradient, is a phase-encoding gradient; G_z, the z-gradient, is a slice-selection gradient. The actual shape and position of these gradients change significantly for different sequences, and their actual makeup is important to field service engineers when performing routine maintenance and troubleshooting for malfunctions.

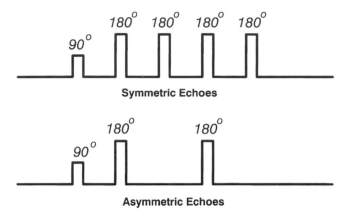

Figure 6–3. For sufficiently long TR values, multiple refocusing pulses can be applied to obtain multiple echoes in either a symmetric or asymmetric manner.

Fast spin-echo imaging is a method of producing spin-echo images in a relatively short period of time. As we will discuss in the next chapter, the time that it takes to complete a scan is determined by the TR, the number of signal averages and the number of phase-encoding steps. Changing the TR will change the character of the scan, which is not an acceptable method of decreasing the time. Decreasing the number of signal averages or decreasing the number of phase-encoding steps will decrease the SNR and the resolution, which are also steps to be avoided. During normal spin-echo imaging, one rf pulse is used for one phase-encoding step. Fast spin-echo techniques make use of an "echo train," in which multiple refocusing (180°) pulses are used during each rf pulse to obtain data for multiple phase-encoding steps from a single rf pulse. If an echo train of 16 is used, for example, then data for 16 phase-encoding steps is obtained from each rf pulse and the total time is approximately 1/16th of the time that the same parameters would take during normal spin-echo imaging. A TR of 3,000 ms and 256-by-128 matrix with two signal averages would normally take 13 minutes. With an echo train of 16, this same scan would only take less than one minute.

The advantage of time is offset by several disadvantages with this technique. Because imaging times are so short, the number of signal averages can be increased to improve the SNR,

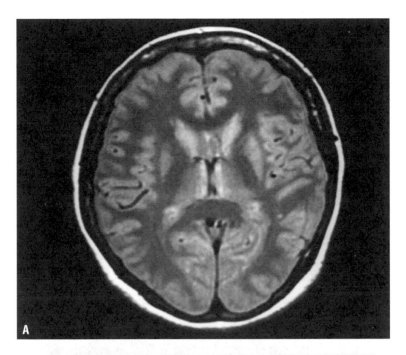

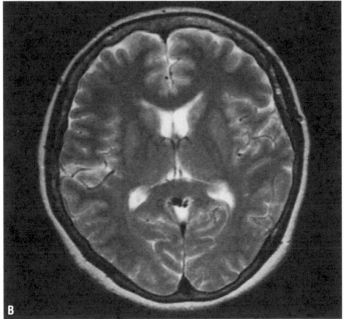

Figure 6–4.   An axial image of the head: (A) TR = 2,000 ms, TE = 20 ms; (B) TR = 2,000 ms, TE = 80 ms.

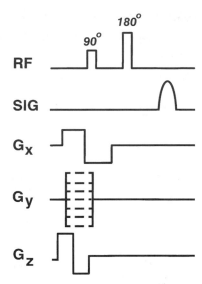

Figure 6–5.   Timing diagram for a simple spin-echo sequence. Time increases as one moves toward the right. The line labeled RF indicates when the 90° and 180° pulses are applied; SIG indicates when the signal is obtained, at a time TE, after the 90° pulse is applied, and at time TE/2, after the application of the 180° pulse; G_x represents the frequency-encoding gradient; G_y represents the phase-encoding gradient, and G_z, the slice-selection gradient.

and the matrix size (number of phase-encoding steps) can be increased to improve resolution. The actual TE is different for each phase-encoding step; however, this is compensated for by applying steeper or more shallow phase-encoding gradients at different points in the scan. Inherently, the contrast between tissues is not as great in this imaging process as with regular spin-echo studies. In addition, the number of slices available is decreased. Increasing the TR increases both the number of slices and the image contrast.

Inversion recovery (IR) sequences produce heavily T1-weighted images using a different pulse sequence than spin-echo techniques. As shown in Figure 6–6, IR images are obtained by first applying a 180° pulse; then after a time TI (inversion time), a 90° pulse is applied, followed by a 180° refocusing pulse. IR images use long TR values with TI times usually between 500 and 800 ms, and very short TEs (10–20 ms). These

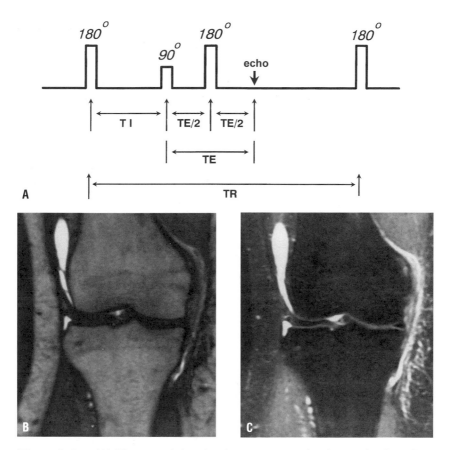

Figure 6–6. (A) Diagram of the rf pulses necessary for the production of an inversion recovery image. Initially a 180° pulse is applied, followed by a 90° pulse at the inversion time (TI). A refocusing, or rephasing, 180° pulse is applied at time TE/2, and the signal is obtained at time TE after the 90° pulse. (B) An inversion recovery image of the knee. (C) A STIR image through the same section as in B, in which the fat signal has been suppressed.

studies can be quite lengthy, unless fast inversion-recovery techniques, exactly comparable to fast spin-echo sequences, are used.

An offshoot of IR imaging, STIR (short TI inversion recovery) imaging is used to eliminate signal from fat. A short TI value, usually 150–170 ms, depending upon field strength, is used. This is the time that corresponds to the point when fat flips from the initial 180° pulse exactly 90° into the transverse plane. Applying a 90° pulse at this time means that there is no component of fat in the transverse plane, and therefore no signal from the fat. This technique is especially valuable when looking for subtle lesions in regions in which large amounts of fat may obscure the abnormality, such as in bone or in the orbits.

Gradient-echo imaging is a method of obtaining "fast scans" and employs variable flip angles of less than 90°. When this is done, only part of the longitudinal magnetization is converted into transverse magnetization (Figure 6–7). Since the signal depends upon the amount of transverse magnetization, the

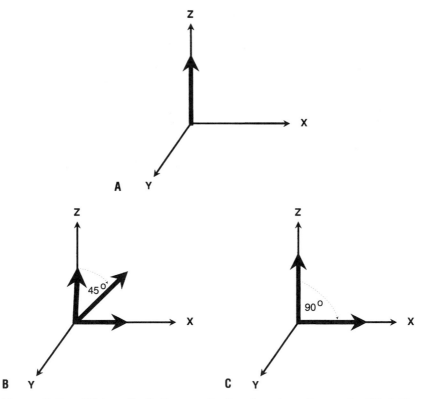

Figure 6–7.   (A) Longitudinal magnetization lies along the *z* axis. (B) A flip angle less than 90° produces transverse magnetization in the *xy* plane, which is of a smaller magnitude than the original longitudinal magnetization. (C) A flip angle of 90° produces transverse magnetization in the *xy* plane, which is exactly equal to the original longitudinal magnetization.

signal eventually obtained will be less than for spin-echo imaging, but it can be acquired more rapidly. To further speed up the imaging process, a gradient rather than a 180° pulse is used for rephasing, because it is faster. If a magnetic gradient is applied to a system, as shown in Figure 6–8, the spins at the higher field end (point A) will have a higher frequency than those at the low frequency end (point B). Assuming that the field is kept on for 2 ms, if the field is reversed the atoms at point B now are at the higher end and spin faster than the atoms at the low end, point A, and after the field has been applied for exactly 2 ms, the spins should be focused again.

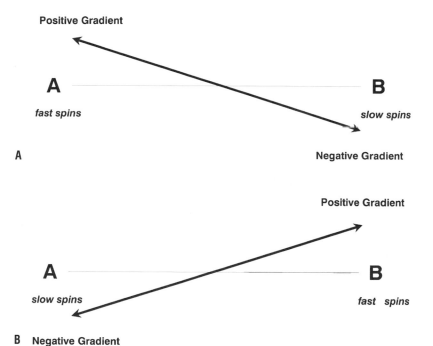

Figure 6–8.   (A) A gradient will change the frequency of precession of spins, with the larger gradients producing faster spins. (B) If the gradient is reversed and maintained for the same time as in A, the effect will be to bring all spins back to the same frequency. Refocusing to form an echo is accomplished with the use of gradients rather than a 180° pulse.

The lack of a 180° pulse increases the effect of field inhomogeneity, and so T2* effects increase significantly. Gradient echo images are also obtained one slice at a time. In spin-echo and inversion-recovery imaging, one pixel on each slice is sequentially obtained, so that no image is completed until the last round of data acquisition. Since the gradient echo images are obtained one slice at a time and are produced very quickly, it is possible to obtain single sections by asking patients to hold their breath and thus minimize the effects of respiratory motion. Another important difference between gradient and spin-echo imaging is that the lack of a 180° pulse allows flowing blood to produce a signal, no matter which slice they happen to be in at the time. Rather than produce a "flow void," or lack of signal in blood vessels, gradient-echo images produce bright signals from vascular structures (Figure 6–9).

MRI studies have long been able to image and identify blood vessels without the use of intravenous injections, because

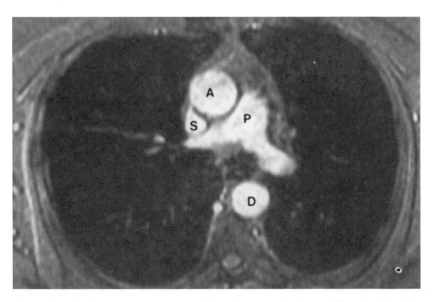

Figure 6–9.   Gradient-echo image through the mid-thorax. Flowing blood is observed to be bright in the ascending aorta (A), the descending aorta (D), the superior vena cava (S), and the main pulmonary trunk (P), which bifurcates into the right and left main pulmonary arteries.

flowing blood presents as regions of absent signal, usually referred to as a "flow void." Blood vessels can be identified by their tubular shape and characteristic lack of signal. As blood is flowing through a vessel, there are usually very few atoms within the slice being imaged that receive both the excitation and rephasing pulses necessary to produce a signal. Since little or no signal is produced, the region is observed as a very dark region on the image (Figure 6–10). In fact, then, MRI depicts soft tissues and can visualize blood vessels because they do not produce an image. Artifacts that cause exceptions to this flow void are discussed in Chapter 9.

During recent years, new types of MR scanning techniques have been developed for clinical examinations to obtain signal from flowing blood and to minimize the signal produced by other structures. These techniques are referred to as magnetic

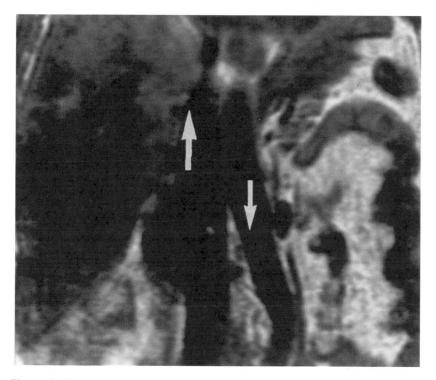

Figure 6–10.   Spin-echo image in which flowing blood (arrows) does not produce a signal.

resonance angiography, or MRA. There are two basic types of MRA: time-of-flight techniques and phase-contrast techniques. Each relies on a completely different set of principles to produce the images; each has certain advantages and disadvantages; each is better used in certain clinical situations; but each method produces the type of images that we refer to as angiograms, without the need for injections or ionizing radiation.

Time-of-flight techniques employ a variation of the principles that were outlined in Chapter 4. The basic premise is that the contrast in the image will be provided by fully relaxed materials (flowing blood with no prior excitations) that enter into a volume, or anatomic slice, in which motionless materials produce a minimal signal. The signal from blood flowing into the section becomes higher than the signal from stationary tissues.

As in spin-echo imaging, the signal from tissues is proportional to the measured transverse magnetization, M_{xy}. The transverse magnetization is created by an rf pulse that rotates the longitudinal magnetization, M_z, into the xy plane. The angle applied, the flip angle, is 90° for spin-echo imaging, but it is significantly shorter for time-of-flight angiography. The greater the flip angle, the larger the transverse magnetization produced, and the larger the signal. The shorter the flip angle, the smaller the signal, but the faster the material can achieve relaxation. Initially, before the first rf pulse is applied, the tissues within the slice have a maximum longitudinal magnetization, M_z^0, which depends upon the concentration of mobile hydrogen atoms and the magnetic field strength. During a short TR pulse, the longitudinal magnetization decreases. After the pulse, the longitudinal magnetization begins to increase. Before it can reach its original value, M_z^0, a second rf pulse is applied quickly (definition of a short TR). This pulse decreases the longitudinal magnetization once again, but this time the starting point is lower. The process is repeated multiple times: an rf pulse decreases the longitudinal magnetization; the longitudinal magnetization begins to increase during relaxation until the next rf pulse is applied. Eventually, a steady-state situation is reached (Figure 6–11) whereby the increase gained during relaxation equals the decrease lost due to the rf pulse, and the value of the longitudinal magnetization remains essentially constant. The value of M_z

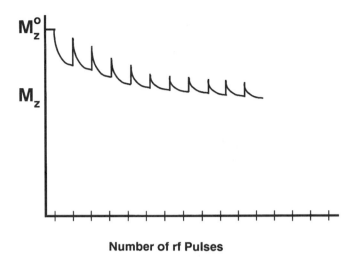

Number of rf Pulses

Figure 6–11. The longitudinal magnetization, M_z, begins with a value of M_x^0. An rf pulse is applied and the longitudinal magnetization begins to decrease. Before it has decreased too far, the rf pulse is stopped and M_z begins to increase. Before it has increased too much, another rf pulse is applied and M_z decreases again. This process is continually repeated. With the proper choice of TR and flip angle, the curve evens out as it approaches a steady state.

at the steady state depends upon the repetition time, the flip angle, and the T1 value of the tissue. The TR and the flip angle are chosen so that the total signal produced by the stationary tissue is minimal.

Blood flowing into the section is not at a steady state and will produce a bright signal, relative to the saturated stationary tissues. The faster the flow of the blood, the further into the slice, or slab, the blood will penetrate before it reaches a steady state and produces the same minimal signal that the stationary tissues do (since the T1 and proton density of blood are very similar to most soft tissues) (Figure 6–12).

Time-of-flight MR angiography can be acquired in essentially two different ways: using two-dimensional acquisition or three-dimensional acquisition. Two-dimensional time-of-flight (2D-TOF) utilizes conventional two-dimensional gradient-echo

BLOOD FLOW

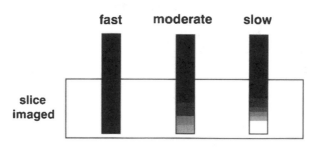

Figure 6–12. Since blood entering a slice is not at a steady state equilibrium, it will produce a positive signal. As soon as the blood enters the slice, it begins to approach a steady state, at which point it will no longer produce a signal. The faster the blood flows, the deeper it will penetrate into the slice before it stops producing a signal.

pulse sequences using flow compensation. The flow-related enhancement is used to distinguish moving from stationary signals. Blood flow into the imaged section will be brighter than stationary molecules. Short repetition times relative to normal tissue T1 values are used to minimize tissue signal and provide maximum vascular contrast enhancement. Signal increases with flow rate to a maximum enhancement at moderate flow. Acquisition times are relatively short (5–7 min). Potential clinical applications include demonstration of the carotid bifurcation, basilar artery occlusive disease, pelvic and lower extremity venous thrombi, and intracranial venous thrombosis. Potential disadvantages include an insensitivity to in-plane flow states, the necessity for thin slices, the possibility of increased false-positive diagnoses for stenoses, and simulated flow-related enhancement in hematomas.

Three-dimensional time-of-flight (3D-TOF) uses conventional three-dimensional gradient-echo pulse sequences and has several advantages over 2D-TOF. Signal-to-noise is significantly increased, very thin sections are possible, and there is an increased sensitivity to moderate and rapid flow rates. This technique provides a high spatial resolution, relatively short scan times, and the ability to utilize very short echo times. Potential clinical applications include evaluation of carotid occlusive disease, intracranial aneurysms, AVM arterial supply, and, using contrast, imaging of venous angiomas. This method suffers from a relative insensitivity to slow flow and is effective for relatively small three-dimensional volumes. Due to the insensitivity to slow flow, this method is unreliable in imaging venous anatomy. "Black blood" angiograms were developed in order to overcome signal loss, leading to an overestimation of stenoses. This technique is essentially a TOF technique in which arterial blood flowing into the slice is presaturated below the region of interest. Minimum-intensity projection angiograms prepared in this manner may permit a more accurate evaluation of stenoses.

In time-of-flight techniques, the farther into the slice the blood flows, the closer the atoms come to reaching steady state; the signal weakens and eventually disappears. In order to minimize artifacts produced by this effect, a variation of the usual 3D-TOF technique is used, called multiple overlapping thick slab angiography (MOTSA). As shown in Figure 6–13, a series of thick slabs are obtained, which overlap each other, usually 25% on both the top and bottom. These slabs are then combined to

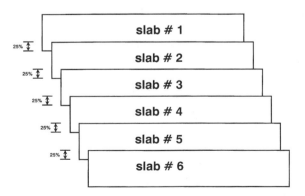

Figure 6–13.   Multiple overlapping thick-slab angiography (MOTSA). Each slab overlaps adjacent slabs by 25%.

produce a volume image that eliminates the decrease in signal with depth of penetration of the blood flow. The overlapping stacking of these slabs produces a characteristic "venetian blind" artifact (Figure 6–14).

The second type of MRA data acquisition is called **phase-contrast imaging**. In this technique, only signal from flowing blood is obtained, with no signal from stationary tissues. Phase-contrast angiography is a quantitative technique, which can be used to determine actual flow velocities. This procedure is based upon a bipolar gradient. Bipolar means that the gradient has a positive and a negative part. In essence, a gradient is applied to a given voxel in two parts: first a positive gradient is applied, and then an equal but opposite negative gradient is applied. Since the positive gradient is the same size as the negative gradient, they cancel each other out, and tissue within the voxel does not experience any effect at all and does not produce a signal.

In order to use this principle for imaging flowing blood, the size of the positive and negative gradients is different for each voxel. Figure 6–15 shows what happens to blood flowing from

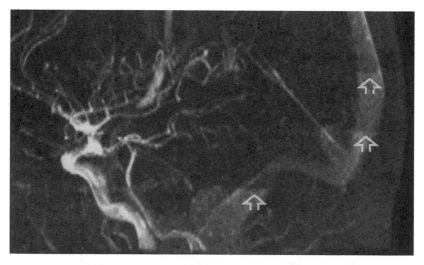

Figure 6–14. Venetian blind artifact in a MOTSA scan of the head. Arrows indicate areas of overlap.

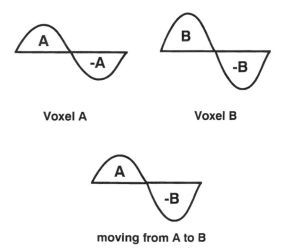

Figure 6–15. Bipolar gradients. At voxel A, first a positive A gradient is applied, followed by a negative A gradient, for a net change of zero to all tissues in the voxel. At voxel B, a positive B gradient is followed by a negative B gradient, also giving a net change of zero for all tissues in the voxel. If blood is flowing in voxel A when the positive gradient is applied, then Is In voxel B when the negative gradient is applied, there is a net nonzero change to the blood since the magnitude of these gradients is different; thus a signal is produced.

voxel A to voxel B while the gradient is applied. All of the stationary tissue in voxel A experiences a positive A gradient and a negative A gradient: they cancel each other out, and stationary tissue in voxel A gives no signal. All of the stationary tissue in voxel B experiences a positive B gradient and a negative B gradient: they cancel each other out, and stationary tissue in voxel B gives no signal. The blood is in voxel A while the positive gradient is applied, but has moved to voxel B when the negative gradient is applied. As seen in the diagram, the positive and negative gradients to the blood are *not* the same: there is a net gradient applied to the blood and the flowing blood produces a signal. If the gradient is made larger and larger the farther away each voxel is, faster-flowing blood experiences a larger difference in gradients and produces a brighter signal. In analyzing this information, flow velocities can be measured. Figure 6–16 is an example of a phase-contrast angiogram of an arteriovenous malformation in the foot.

Three-dimensional phase contrast (3D-PC) techniques rely on velocity-induced phase shifts in order to differentiate flowing blood from stationary tissues. It can be sensitive to slow flow in small vessels because phase shift is due to flowing blood and offers the potential of quantitative measurements of blood velocity. Velocity encoding permits selection of variable velocities. Signal-to-noise ratio is higher than from 2D-PC, and this method has the ability to suppress backgrounds. Large volumes can be imaged, both arterial and venous structures can be imaged, and both magnitude and phase images can be generated. Potential clinical applications include evaluation of AVMs, intracranial aneurysms, venous malformations and occlusions, congenital abnormalities, and traumatic vascular injuries. Disadvantages include relatively long imaging times and a sensitivity to signal loss from turbulent flow; in addition, pre-evaluation with 2D-PC may be required to determine the optimal value for velocity encoding.

Two-dimensional phase contrast (2D-PC) studies utilize bipolar phase-encoding gradients similar to that of 3D-PC, except that a series of two-dimensional sections are obtained and projected as a single two-dimensional plane. Flow compensation is unnecessary, so that echo time can be decreased, thus shortening imaging time. This quicker scan permits one to vary the velocity-encoding parameters over a wide range, so that emphasis can be shifted from arterial to venous structures relatively easily. Potential clinical applications include use as a localizing scan before 3D-PC, detecting slow-flow states in AVMs and aneurysms, and assessing portal vein anatomy and flow states. Disadvantages include the inability to obtain multiple projections, retrospectively, and a necessity for a relatively large voxel size, resulting in diminished resolution.

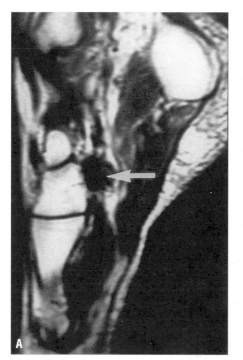

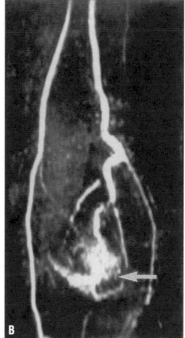

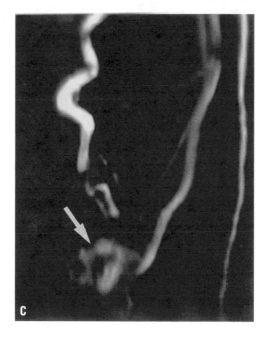

Figure 6–16. (A) Spin-echo image of an arteriovenous malformation (arrow) in the foot. (B) 3D-TOF angiogram of the same arteriovenous malformation. (C) The same pathology imaged using phase-contrast techniques.

POINTS TO PONDER

- Pulse sequences are combinations of rf pulses designed to produce an image.

- The most commonly used pulse sequences are spin-echo, gradient-echo, fast spin-echo, and inversion-recovery techniques.

- Spin-echo images are produced by exciting the atoms with a 90° rf pulse, then rephasing (refocusing) their signal using a 180° rf pulse.

- T1-weighted images have high resolution and low contrast.

- T2-weighted images have high contrast and lower resolution.

- Fast spin-echo imaging uses an "echo train": multiple refocusing pulses that produce multiple phase-encoding steps from one rf pulse.

- Gradient-echo images are fast scans that use a flip angle of less than 90°.

- MR angiography uses either time-of-flight or phase-contrast techniques.

- Time-of-flight techniques rely on stationary tissues achieving a steady-state equilibrium and producing a minimum signal. Only flowing blood will then be bright.

- The faster blood flows in time-of-flight techniques, the deeper it will penetrate while giving a signal.

- MOTSA (multiple overlapping thick-slab angiography) techniques eliminate the decrease in signal from a vessel as it penetrates into a section.

- Phase-contrast techniques employ equal positive and negative gradients for each voxel but a different value for different voxels.

- The equal positive and negative gradients cancel out for stationary tissues so they do not produce a signal.

- Flowing blood experiences a different positive and negative gradient, since it is moving through different voxels, and will produce a bright signal.

SCANNING PARAMETERS AND TECHNIQUES

Setting up an MRI scan involves making decisions about many parameters, each of which affects the quality of the scan. The most important of these choices is the pulse sequence. T1- or T2 weighted spin-echo, gradient-echo, inversion-recovery, or vascular sequences produce vastly different images and provide different types of anatomic and pathologic information. Within each pulse sequence, a multitude of choices must be made, with each parameter potentially able to affect the appearance of the images radically.

Initially, the operator must enter patient data: name, sex, age, weight, type of examination, and so on. The operator then designates positioning and equipment parameters. Method of entry (head or feet first), position of the patient (supine, prone, or decubitus), and type of coil (head coil, body coil, or surface coil) are entered by observing how the patient was placed in the unit and which type of coil is being used. Fundamental decisions must be made in advance as to the pulse sequence to be employed and the imaging plane desired. These choices depend upon the part of the body being imaged and the information desired. Once the initial anatomic plane is decided upon, a landmark is established. This involves marking the center of the area of interest as the zero point (center of reference) from which all subsequent scans are planned. The first imaging plane chosen is often referred to as a **scout image**. Sometimes this is a rapidly achieved, low-resolution gradient-echo image, whose sole purpose is to establish anatomic landmarks (Figure 7–1). Although these images can be obtained in one minute or less, a high-quality T1-weighted spin-echo image takes about two minutes and yields excellent anatomic (and sometimes pathologic) information (Figure 7–2). It has been our experience that the fast, low-resolution scout images are a waste of time; thus we use high-resolution T1-weighted images as a "scout" for all studies. In the long run we find that time is actually saved and more information is acquired by using this technique.

Multiple parameters that are common to all pulse sequences must be selected while setting up the scanning sequence, each of

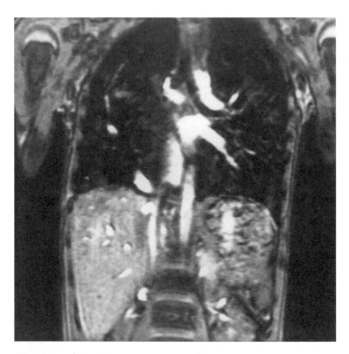

Figure 7–1. Coronal gradient-echo scout, showing anatomic structures but no useful clinical information. Scan was obtained in 53 seconds.

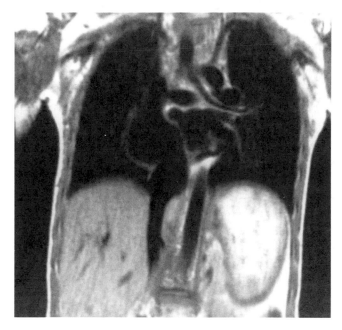

Figure 7–2. Coronal spin-echo image with significant anatomic detail obtained in 1 minute, 32 seconds.

which can significantly alter the appearance of the image. These include the slice thickness, interslice spacing, field of view, number of signal averages, matrix size, scan location, bandwidth, echo time, and repetition time. Additional pulse-sequence-specific parameters, such as flip angle, inversion time, and saturation pulses, must be selected when required.

The proper combination of these parameters is essential to obtain the best possible study. It should always be remembered that the best possible study is not necessarily obtained by choosing the parameters that will permit the maximum resolution. Theoretically, the resolution of a scan can be improved in several ways, most easily by increasing the matrix size and the number of signal averages. The effect of these changes, however, can drastically affect the imaging time. The time required for a spin-echo sequence is given by the equation

$$\text{Time} = \text{TR} \cdot N_{ex} \cdot \text{PE}$$

where TR is the repetition time, N_{ex} is the number of signal averages, and PE represents the number of phase-encoding steps.

A compromise must be made between resolution and time. Although high resolution should be strived for, if scanning time is too long it becomes less economically feasible. In addition, the longer the time for a single scan, the greater the probability that the patient will move, thus degrading the resolution with motion artifact.

The number of signal averages, also referred to as the number of excitations, is the number of times a signal is obtained from each voxel. As discussed previously, in addition to the signal from the tissue within each voxel, noise is inherent in the imaging process. This means that extraneous signal from noise will contaminate the true signal from the tissue being imaged. If only a single measurement is made, this contamination will change the true appearance of the voxel. If several measurements are made and the values added, the value of the random noise can be minimized. The signal-to-noise ratio (SNR) increases by the square root of the number of signal averages. Therefore, if N_{ex} is doubled, the SNR increases by $\sqrt{2}$, or 1.4. A 100% increase in the N_{ex} will result in only a 40% increase in the SNR. While this is still a significant increase in SNR, large values of N_{ex} will not significantly increase resolution, as shown in Table 7–1 for a typical two-minute scan.

There is definitely a diminishing return in increasing the SNR by increasing the number of signal averages. Raising the

TABLE 7–1. SIGNAL AVERAGE EFFECTS ON SNR AND TIME

Number of Signal Averages	Relative Signal-to-Noise Ratio	Relative Time
1	1	2 min
2	1.4	4 min
3	1.7	6 min
4	2	8 min
8	2.8	16 min
10	3.1	20 min

N_{ex} from 1 to 10 increases scanning time from 2 to 20 minutes, but it increases SNR only about three times. Increasing from 1 N_{ex} to 2 N_{ex} improves the image, but the slight further increase in resolution brought about by an increase to 10 N_{ex} is rarely worth the extra 16 minutes of scanning time. If this were a long TR scan with an imaging time of 8 minutes at 2 N_{ex}, a 10 N_{ex} scan would take 40 minutes. Figure 7–3 shows the increased resolution due to increased N_{ex}.

Noise can also be decreased, and SNR therefore improved, by changing the bandwidth. In theory, we would like each voxel to correspond to a single frequency. In practice, this is not possible. The signal absorbed and emitted by tissue in a single voxel actually has a finite width. In order to assure that the coil can receive as much signal as possible, a bandwidth, representing a range of frequencies, is used. A wide bandwidth includes more noise with the true signal. A narrow bandwidth reduces the amount of noise picked up by the receiver. Although a narrow bandwidth would appear always to be preferable, as was shown in Chapter 4, the sampling time is related to the bandwidth. If the bandwidth is decreased too much, the scanning time and the TE will have to be increased.

Selecting the matrix size, which determines the number of phase-encoding steps, is important in determining the time of the scan, the SNR, and the resolution. It has already been shown (Chapter 2) how the matrix size affects the resolution of an image. The smaller the pixels, the greater the resolution. Small pixels permit the imaging of smaller structures and show greater detail. However, the trade-off in this case is that if the pixels are too small, they will not contain enough signal and the SNR will be decreased. Increasing the number of pixels in the phase-encoding direction increases the number of phase-encoding steps, and therefore also increases the scanning time. One can obtain a significant increase in resolution by increasing the matrix size, as illustrated in Figures 7–3 and 7–4.

The field of view (FOV) is defined as the size of the scanning area and is given in centimeters. A 24-cm FOV describes a scanning area of 24 cm by 24 cm. The FOV and the matrix permit a calculation of the pixel size:

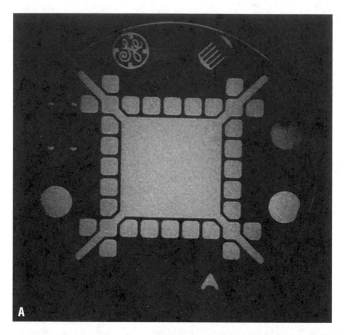

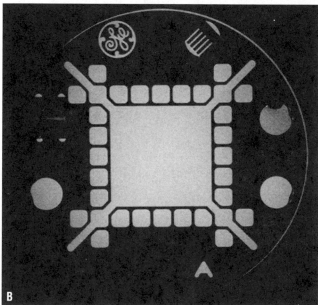

Figure 7–3.   (A) Image of a phantom obtained at 1 N_{ex} and a 256-by-128 matrix. (B) The same section as in A with the N_{ex} increased to 2. Notice the increase in signal intensity and less grainy appearance due to the SNR in B.

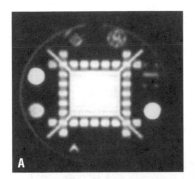

Figure 7–4A. Imaging phantom scanned in the body coil. (A) FOV = 48 cm, TR = 500 ms, TE = 20 ms, 1 N_{ex}. Structures are visible but vague. Signal is high because pixel size is large.

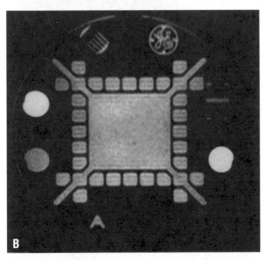

Figure 7–4B. Same section, but the FOV has been decreased to 24 cm, increasing the resolution of structures.

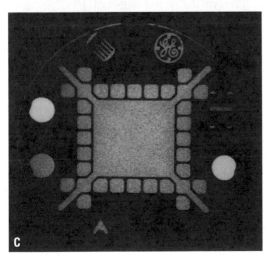

Figure 7–4C. Same section as in B, but matrix size has been increased from 256-by-256 to 512-by-512, further increasing resolution, but decreasing SNR. The grainier appearance is due to a lower signal per pixel, since the pixel sizes are much smaller, but resolution has increased, making details more visible.

Pixel size = FOV/matrix

A matrix of 256-by-128 and an FOV of 24 cm would result in rectangular pixels that in the frequency-encoding direction would be 24/256 = 0.94 mm, and in the phase-encoding direction would be 24/128 = 1.9 mm. A 512-by-512 matrix would result in square pixels, 24/512 = 0.47 mm on a side. Since the number of phase-encoding steps would increase from 128 to 512, the scanning time would have to increase to four times longer in order to obtain this increased resolution. For a given matrix size, the larger the field of view, the larger the pixels and the lower the resolution. Conversely, the smaller the field of view, the smaller the pixel size and the greater the resolution. Figure 7–4 demonstrates the increase in resolution as the FOV is decreased.

The thickness of the slices will affect both the quality of the images and the quality of the interpretations. The thicker the slice, the larger will be the size of the voxel, and the more signal will be contained within it. This combination will give the appearance of a high-resolution image, with an inherently higher SNR. Although the images will be more pleasing to the eye if the slice thickness is increased, too large a slice thickness may conceal important clinical information, as small structures will be combined with overlying structures.

In addition to the thickness of the slice, the spacing between slices has a great bearing on the SNR. As previously noted, the signal exciting a given voxel contains a range of frequencies, rather than a single, discrete frequency. The shape of the signal pulse can vary, but most often it resembles that illustrated in Figure 7–5A. As the figure shows, because of the shape of the signal, part of it lies outside of the slice of interest. If a single-slice acquisition is used, such as is done in gradient-echo pulse sequences, there will be no effect on other slices. In multislice acquisitions, however, as seen in Figure 7–5B, part of the signal exciting slice 1 will overlap into slice 2. This overlap of signal from one slice to another is called **crosstalk**. Crosstalk acts as an extraneous signal source and will significantly increase the noise in a given slice. In order to avoid this problem, rather than have slices too close together, a gap is left between slices, which is referred to as the interslice gap. This gap is wide enough so

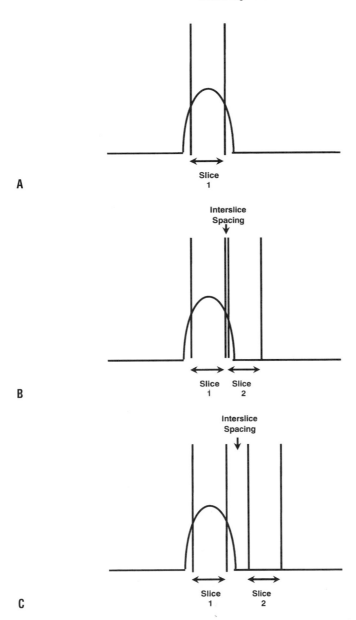

Figure 7–5. (A) The shape of the signal pulse often causes it to extend outside of the slice being imaged. (B) Signal from slice 1 extends into slice 2, where
it is perceived as noise. (C) With a sufficient interslice gap, the signal from slice
1 extends only into the interslice gap and does not interfere with slice 2.

that crosstalk from adjacent slices will fall completely within the gap and will not interfere with other slices (Figure 7–5C). An interslice gap of approximately 50% of the slice thickness is usually considered sufficient to eliminate crosstalk. Figure 7–6 illustrates how crosstalk affects the quality of an image.

Another method of minimizing the effects of crosstalk is to change the shape of the signal pulse so that very little signal overlaps the boundaries of the slice of interest (see Figure 7–7A). Because the crosstalk is minimized, the next slice can be positioned much closer to the first slice, with a smaller interslice gap (Figure 7–7B). By keeping most of the signal within the slice, the change in shape also decreases the height of the pulse so that each voxel receives less signal. This "close-spaced" option is offered on many systems. The decreased signal is usually not sufficient to affect the quality of the images significantly, unless signal from within the voxels is inherently low, as in thin-section, high-resolution views using a large matrix and small FOV.

When it is clinically important to obtain slices that are either very close together, or actually touching so that there is no interslice gap (e.g., high-resolution IAC images or meniscal views of the knee), a technique called **interleaved slices** can be used (Figure 7–8). This technique actually employs two consecutive scans, the first obtaining data from the even-numbered slices and the second from the odd-numbered slices. This means that the interslice gap is equal to 100% of the slice thickness, so that there is no interference from crosstalk. The scan time is doubled using this technique, since two separate scans are actually performed. In considering this option, it is important to appreciate the difference between two usually interchangeable terms: contiguous and interleaved. The interleaved option obtains adjacent slices with no gaps by employing two scans with large interslice gaps; the images do not have any interference from crosstalk. **Contiguous slices** also produce adjacent slices with no gaps, but they are obtained in a single scan with a zero gap; there will be effects from crosstalk. Interleaved slices take twice as long to obtain as contiguous slices. Figure 7–6 illustrates the difference in image quality between these two techniques.

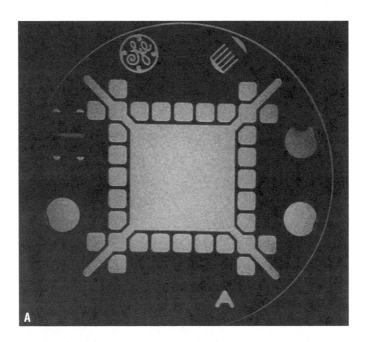

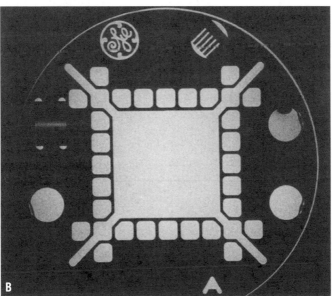

Figure 7–6. (A) Image of a phantom where slices were contiguous and crosstalk decreased SNR. (B) Same section as in A, where images were obtained using an interleaved technique.

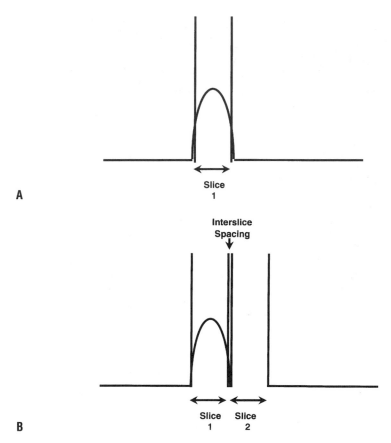

Figure 7–7. (A) Signal pulse has a different shape than those observed in Figure 7–5 and barely extends outside of the slice. Note that total signal strength (equal to the area under the curve) is less than that in Figure 7–5. (B) Slices can be positioned closer together without crosstalk affecting the images.

The repetition time, TR, and the echo time, TE, are the two parameters that have the largest effect on the appearance of the image. For spin-echo imaging, the shorter the TR and TE values, the more T1 weighted the image will be; the longer the TR and TE values, the more T2 weighted the image will be. These parameters are also inherently involved in the determination of the SNR (Figures 7–9 and 7–10). TR is the length of time that is allowed to pass before the next rf pulse is applied. Since the longitudinal magnetization begins to recover after the application

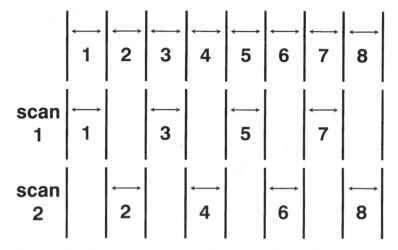

Figure 7–8. Interleaved technique. If adjacent slices 1–8 are required, as in the top row, two consecutive scans are performed. The first scan images the odd-numbered slices, leaving a 100% interslice gap, and the second scan images the even-numbered slices in a similar manner.

of the initial rf pulse, there will have been more longitudinal recovery for longer TRs, and therefore there will be more magnetization available to be flipped into the transverse plane when the next rf pulse is applied. This means that the signal will be stronger and the SNR will increase. If the TR is very short, not all of the longitudinal magnetization will have recovered, less will be available to be flipped at the next rf pulse, and the signal will be weaker. Figure 7–11 depicts the signal obtained from substances with both long and short T1 values at a short TR and at a long TR. At short TR values, there will be a larger contribution from tissues with short T1 values; at long TR values, a greater signal will be obtained from material with both long and short T1 values.

The echo time, TE, also affects the SNR. As illustrated in Chapter 4, transverse magnetization produces the MR signal. TE determines how long after the rf pulse the signal is collected. Since transverse magnetization begins to decay as soon as the rf pulse stops, the longer the TE, the less the transverse magnetization left in the xy plane to produce a signal. Shorter TE values

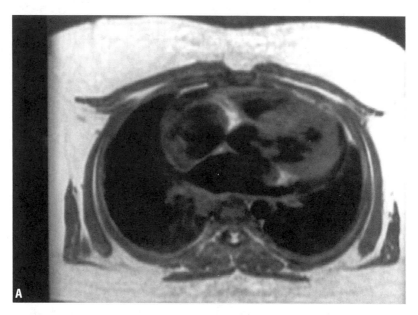

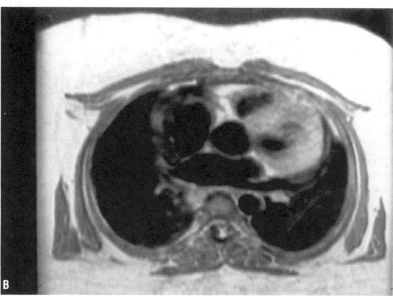

Figure 7–9.   (A) T1-weighted image through the heart of a patient who suffered a recent myocardial infarction, with TR = 700 ms and TE = 20 ms. (B) The same anatomic section with TR = 2,100 ms and TE = 20 ms. SNR is higher than in A because of the increased signal due to the higher TR. While fat remains bright on both images, note the brighter signal in the myocardium of the left ventricle in image B due to edema in the cardiac muscle after the infarction.

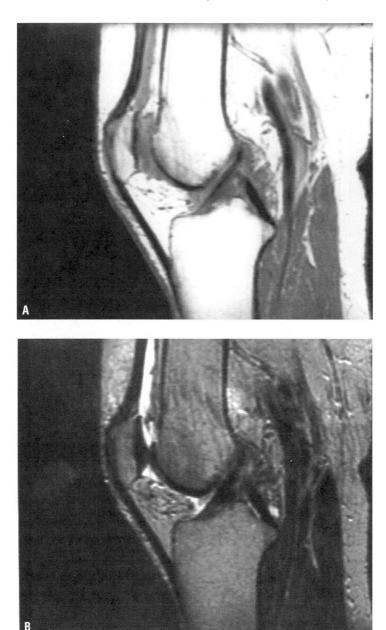

Figure 7–10.   (A) Section through the knee with TR = 1,500 ms and TE = 20 ms. High-resolution proton density image with high SNR. (B) Same section with TR = 1,500 ms and TE = 80 ms. This T2-weighted image has higher contrast, but lower SNR due to increased TE. Note decrease in signal from both fat and muscle on the longer TE image B.

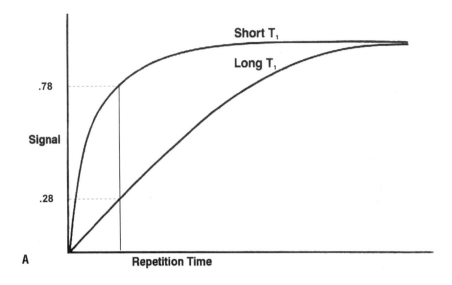

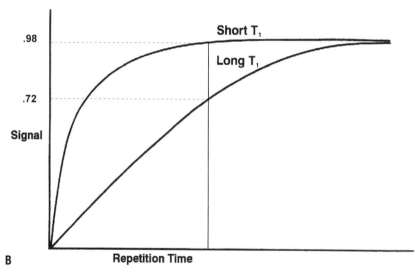

Figure 7–11. Graph of signal intensity changes as a function of repetition time. (A) If a short repetition time is used, the short T1 tissue will have a relative signal intensity of 0.78, while the long T1 tissue will have a relative intensity of 0.28. (B) If the TR is lengthened, the signal intensity of the short T1 material increases to 0.98, while that of the long T1 material increases to 0.72. All signals increase with a longer TR. The relative brightness of tissues with short T1 values is increased by using a shorter TR.

will produce more signal, and therefore a higher SNR; longer TE values will produce less signal and a lower SNR. Figure 7–12 illustrates how different TE values affect the signal from both high T2 and low T2 tissues.

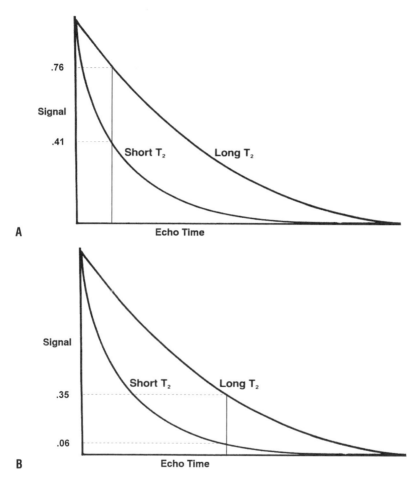

Figure 7–12. Graph of signal intensity changes as a function of echo time. (A) If a short TE is used, material with a short T2 will have a relative signal intensity of 0.41, and that of a long T2 tissue will be 0.76. (B) If the TE is increased, the short T2 material signal drops to 0.06 and the signal from the long T2 tissue drops to 0.35. Increasing the TE decreases the total signal and will therefore decrease SNR. The relative brightness of tissues with long T2 values is increased by using a longer TE.

There are a great number of parameters that can be altered in order to produce an MR image. Each will change the quality of the image in a variety of ways, which are summarized in Table 7–2. Resolution and SNR can always be increased at the expense of increasing the scanning time, and a compromise has to be reached. The compromise will often be different in different situations, and the clinical question, the status of the patient, and nature of the study will be important factors in the choice of the final imaging parameters utilized.

TABLE 7–2. SCANNING PARAMETER EFFECT ON IMAGE ACQUISITION

Parameter	Value	SNR	Resolution	Scanning Time
TR	High	↑	↑	↑
	Low	↓	↓	↓
N_{ex}	High	↑	↑	↑↑
	Low	↓	↓	↓
Matrix	High	↓	↑↑	↑
	Low	↑	↓↓	↓
FOV	Large	↑	↓	–
	Small	↓	↑	–
Slice thickness	Thick	↑	↓	–
	Thin	↓	↑	–
Slice spacing	Narrow	↓	↓	–
	Wide	↑	↑	–
Bandwidth	Narrow	↑	↑	↑
	Wide	↓	↓	↓

POINTS TO PONDER

- Multiple parameters will determine the appearance of an MR image.

- Most parameters that will increase resolution and SNR will also cause an increase in scanning time.

- Scanning time will depend upon the TR, the N_{ex}, and the number of phase-encoding steps in the image matrix.

- The SNR will increase as the square root of the increase in number of signal averages.

- Decreasing the bandwidth will also decrease the noise (and raise the SNR) but may cause an increase in the scanning time and raise the minimum TE.

- Image resolution will be prominently affected by an increase in the matrix size, which will also cause an increase in the scanning time.

- Decreasing the field of view (FOV) will cause pixel size to be smaller and result in an increased resolution.

- Pixel size is equal to the FOV divided by the matrix size.

- An interslice gap of sufficient magnitude must be maintained in order to prevent increased noise from crosstalk.

- Crosstalk can also be prevented by using signal pulses of different shapes or by interleaving slices.

- Increasing TR will increase signal and increase SNR.

- Increasing TE will decrease signal and decrease SNR.

CHAPTER EIGHT

SPECIAL PROCEDURES AND TECHNIQUES

Many techniques are available to complement the standard pulse sequences which enable overcoming certain problems, or obtaining specific data in certain cases. For example, there are several techniques that will minimize or reorient the unwanted effects of physiologic motion and blood flow, decrease scanning time with a minimum of lost resolution for anxious patients, or even eliminate signal from protons found in fat or in water. Of these many different procedures, the most often used and most important involve minimizing the effects of cardiac and respiratory motion.

CARDIAC GATING

The beating of the heart can cause significant motion artifacts on an MR image, which will cause a blurring of the structures. While this blurring cannot always be eliminated, it can be significantly minimized by using a procedure called **electrocardiogram (ECG) gating** (Figure 8–1). The electrical impulses that cause the normal cycle of cardiac contraction (Figure 8–2)

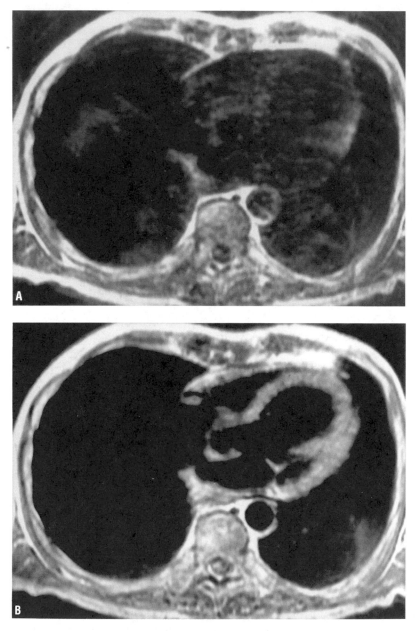

Figure 8–1. Axial sections through the heart. (A) Non-cardiac gated. (B) Cardiac gated. Both sections represent the same anatomic level. Notice the exceptional increase in resolution in the gated image.

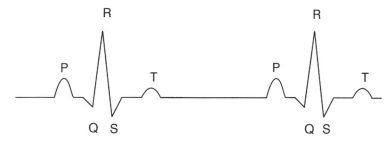

Figure 8–2. The normal electrocardiogram (ECG). The P wave represents contraction of the atria, the QRS complex represents systole (contraction of the ventricles), and the T wave represents the filling of the atria.

produce a series of waves, which correspond to the various motions in the pulsating heart. These deviations from a straight line are indicated by letters P through T (sometimes U). The P wave is caused by the voltage causing the contraction of both the left and right atrium; the QRS complex occurs as both of the ventricles contract; and the T wave indicates a period of recovery during which the left atrium fills with blood from the pulmonary veins and the right atrium fills with blood from the inferior and the superior vena cavae. Of these peaks, the R wave is the most prominent and is much higher than any of the others. Because it is so much higher than the other waves, the R wave can easily be identified electronically. The R wave serves as the "trigger," or starting point, for the rf pulse. An rf pulse is emitted every time an R wave is detected electronically. Since the TR is the time between rf pulses, the TR is thus determined by the patient's heart rate (Figure 8–3). For longer TR values—if a T2-weighted study is required, for example—the system can be set to emit an rf pulse every second, third, or fourth R wave that is recorded (Figure 8–4).

Unlike noncardiac gated spin-echo scans, the entire TR interval cannot be used for data acquisition purposes. ECG tracings are not always exactly regular, even in the most normal of hearts. The heart rate always varies somewhat, so that the R wave for a given heartbeat may appear slightly earlier than expected. In order to be sure that data is not being collected

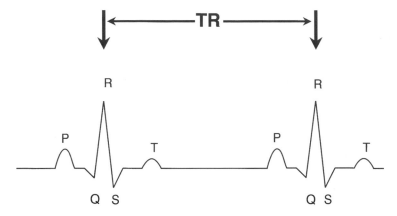

Figure 8–3.   The repetition time (TR) is determined by the heart rate and is defined as the time between successive R waves. At each R wave, an rf pulse is produced.

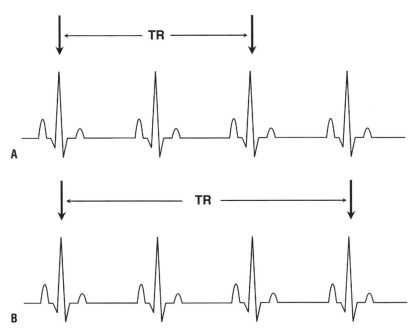

Figure 8–4.   In order to increase the TR, the computer can be programmed to emit the rf pulse every second or third R wave.

when the R wave appears (which will cause it to be "missed" by the computer), a trigger window is chosen (Figure 8–5). This trigger window, usually expressed as a percentage of the R–R interval, is a time at the end of the cardiac cycle, just before the expected R wave is to appear, which is "dead time" as far as scanning is concerned. No data can be collected during this period in order that the R wave may be detected. This shortens the useful length of the repetition time. Since the R wave signals the beginning of systole, the vigorous contraction of the ventricles during which there is maximum cardiac motion, the period right after the R wave is the least appealing for imaging purposes and a trigger delay is used (Figure 8–6). This trigger delay postpones data acquisition for a short time, until cardiac motion has slowed slightly. The combination of the trigger window at one end of the cardiac cycle and the trigger delay at the other limits the useful time available for collecting data (Figure 8–7). This is why fewer slices can be obtained from ECG-gated sequences that appear to have the same TR as a nongated scan.

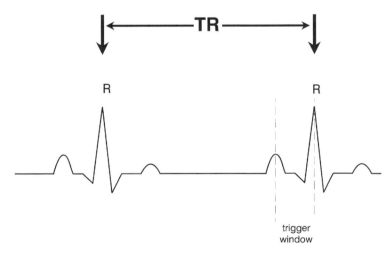

Figure 8–5. The trigger window is the time at the end of the R–R interval during which no data is acquired as the system prepares for the appearance of the next R wave, which will generate another rf pulse.

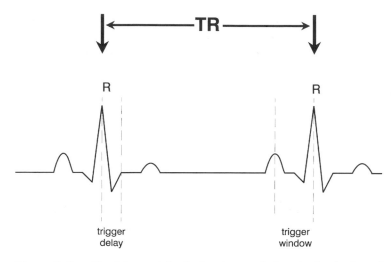

Figure 8–6.   The trigger delay is the time period at the beginning of the R–R interval during which no data is acquired because it is the period of maximum cardiac motion.

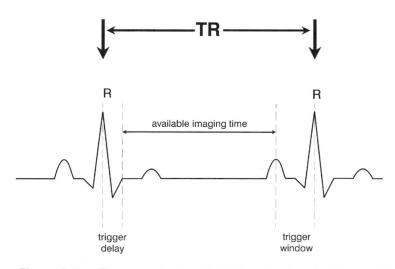

Figure 8–7.   The amount of available imaging time is decreased because of the limitations imposed by the trigger window and trigger delay.

Usually, three or four insulated ECG leads are placed on the patient's back in a pattern determined by the manufacturer to provide the best signal. Since not all patients are alike, it will occasionally require some modification by trial and error to obtain a signal that is strong enough for the system to recognize the R wave. In addition to regular ECG leads, peripheral gating can also be used.

Peripheral gating employs a sensor, which fits around a finger and produces an electrical impulse with every arterial pulsation. This pulsation serves the same purpose as the R wave, in that it acts as the trigger for the rf pulse. The pulse actually occurs approximately 0.2 to 0.3 seconds after the actual R wave, so that the trigger delay and trigger pulse should be adjusted accordingly. Peripheral gating is particularly helpful in patients with arrhythmias, or irregular heart rates, which cause difficulties in obtaining acceptable images.

During nongated scanning procedures, if a single slice is obtained, after the refocusing pulse there is a relatively long period of time during which nothing occurs until the next rf pulse is generated (Figure 8–8). This time can be utilized by starting the next slice selection pulse, then the next, then the next, etc., until it is time for the rf pulse for the first slice to be

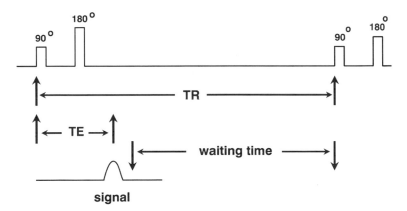

Figure 8–8.   During a single-slice spin-echo sequence, after the data is acquired there is an appreciable time delay before the next rf pulse is generated.

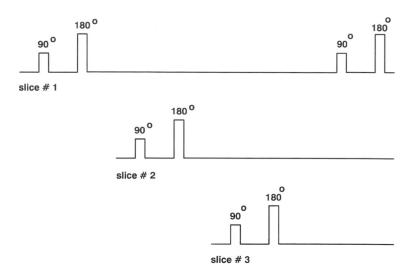

Figure 8–9. A multislice spin-echo sequence utilizes the "waiting time" of a single-slice acquisition to obtain data from additional slices. Since a magnetic gradient has been applied in the slice-selection direction, each slice resonates with a different Larmor frequency, so that there is no interference from imaged slices.

produced (Figure 8–9). The number of slices able to be obtained is determined by the length of the TR. For the same TR value, less time is available for imaging in a cardiac gated scan because of the trigger delay and the trigger window, as seen in Figure 8–7. In addition, although the study is ECG gated, each slice is obtained in a different phase of the cardiac cycle (Figure 8–10). Practically, however, the slices are almost always obtained during the "resting" or diastolic phase of the cardiac cycle when motion is at a minimum. The trigger window and the trigger delay eliminate data acquisition during the systolic phase, when motion (contraction) is at a maximum.

DYNAMIC IMAGING

CINE imaging refers to obtaining images of a moving structure, such as cardiac motion, joint motion (patellar tracking or TMJ mobility), or dynamic flow, and displaying the images in a rapid, continuous loop so that the motion can be observed on

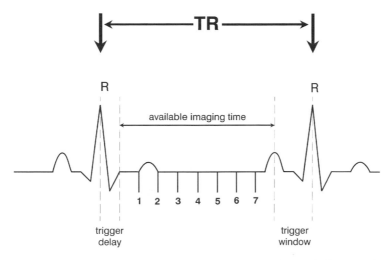

Figure 8–10. During a multislice cardiac-gated acquisition, each image is obtained at a different point of the cardiac cycle. (Location of the images may not be sequential, to minimize cross-talk.)

the display screen. For cardiac imaging, each slice is obtained at multiple phases of the cardiac cycle (Figure 8–11). Spin-echo images can be obtained and replayed in a CINE mode, but only one slice can be obtained at a time, and covering the entire heart would be a very time-consuming process. Gradient-echo images, with their very short repetition and echo times, can acquire multiple slices and multiple phases in relatively short periods of time. The examination is still ECG gated, but since the TR of the gradient-echo images is fixed, the ECG tracing is used only to match the image with the proper phase of the cardiac cycle. After all of the images have been acquired, the images of the different cardiac phases in one single section are played back continuously to produce a dynamic image of the heart.

Joint motion can be observed in a similar manner. An image of the knee or the TMJ is obtained in one position, then the joint is moved a short distance and a second image is obtained. This is repeated until the full range of motion of the joint has been covered. For best results a mechanical device can be used that permits the joint to move an equal prescribed amount between each image. Flow through vessels or the flow of CSF can also be obtained using variations on this technique.

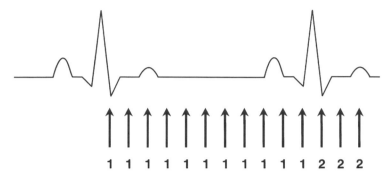

Figure 8–11. CINE cardiac imaging is performed by obtaining the same anatomic section (1) in different phases of the cardiac cycle. This is followed by obtaining a different section (2) in the same manner. Each anatomic section is then viewed in a CINE mode—rapidly viewing the sequential images to produce the appearance of the pulsating heart.

RESPIRATORY CORRECTIONS

Respiratory motion also causes blurring in the imaging of the chest and abdomen. Data acquisition is relatively long in normal spin-echo imaging, so that movement of the chest or abdomen will significantly decrease resolution. The artifact, like all motion-related artifacts, will occur in the phase-encoding direction. One method of modifying the effects of this motion, if it interferes with the interpretation of the image, is to switch the phase- and frequency-encoding directions. The artifact will then be aimed in the opposite direction, and thus out of the area of interest, which will enable the image to be diagnostic (Figure 8–12).

Another way to minimize respiratory artifact is to use one of the fast imaging techniques (gradient-echo, fast spin-echo, spoiled grass, etc.), which decrease imaging time to such a point that breath holding techniques will work. The scanning parameters are set so that pauses during imaging can be anywhere from 6 to 30 seconds (any longer would be impractical). The patient is told to breathe normally, then take a deep breath and hold it for the specified period of time. The scan starts, then stops after a short interval, and the patient is told to breathe normally again. When the patient is ready, the process is repeated until all of the images are obtained. The advantage is that the

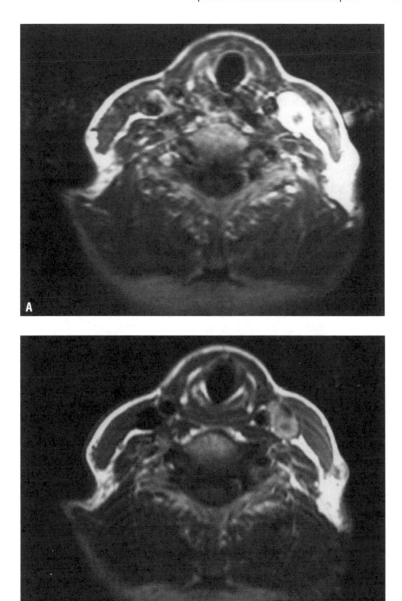

Figure 8–12. (A) Axial image through the neck with the phase-encoding direction left to right. Motion artifact (due to flow in this case) obscures the resolution of the trachea, which was the area of clinical interest. (B) By switching phase and frequency directions, the phase-encoding direction is now anterior to posterior (up and down) and the trachea is well seen.

respiratory motion artifact is essentially eliminated. The disadvantages are that the images obtained have relatively limited contrast, and imaging time is increased because of the time taken during the pauses.

True respiratory gating can be used in a manner similar to that employed in cardiac gating. A belt containing an air-filled bellows is placed around the patient's chest or abdomen (always around the area of imaging interest). A typical respiratory tracing is shown in Figure 8–13. Several disadvantages are inherent in using a true respiratory gating. Respiratory rates are much slower than cardiac rates, so that TR values, the time between respiratory peaks, are much longer, and T1-weighted images are very difficult to obtain. The "peak" in a respiratory tracing is much broader than the R wave in an ECG, so that the "trigger" is less precise. In addition, respiratory rates are much more variable than cardiac rates, and so a precise TR value would be difficult to obtain. Abdominal or chest wall motion is most pronounced at the peaks of the respiratory tracing, so that many techniques only acquire data in the "troughs," where motion is at a minimum (Figure 8–14).

Rather than respiratory gating, the technique used most often to correct for respiratory motion is called **respiratory compensation**. This technique also uses a bellows-type device placed around the patient. As the patient inhales, the chest or abdominal girth increases and stretches the bellows, and the pressure in the bellows decreases. This alteration is translated into an electrical signal that indicates whether the patient is in inspiration or expiration. Rather than acquire the image data in

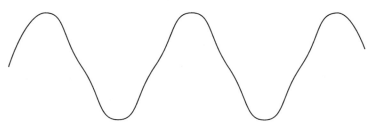

Figure 8–13.   Respiratory tracing is highly variable among individuals, and can vary significantly for an individual as well.

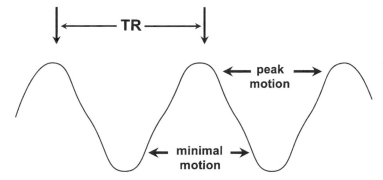

Figure 8–14. The least amount of motion due to respiration is found just after the patient has exhaled (end expiration). There will usually be a short while with no motion before the patient begins to inhale.

the usual manner, there is a reordering of the way in which the data is obtained. Shallow phase-encoding gradients are relatively insensitive to motion, whereas steep phase-encoding gradients produce severe motion artifacts. For this reason, when the computer senses that the patient is in inspiration (maximum motion), the shallow phase-encoding gradients are used to minimize the effect. At minimum motion, during end expiration, steep phase-encoding gradients are used, since there will be little motion to cause artifacts (Figure 8–15). This method uses precise TR values, can produce either T1- or T2-weighted images, and does not increase imaging time while producing images with decreased respiratory artifact (Figure 8–16).

SATURATION PULSES

Another way to minimize respiratory motion is to use properly positioned saturation pulses. A **saturation pulse**, or presaturation pulse, is a 90° pulse applied over an area before the normal 90° saturation pulse is applied. When the 90° excitation pulse is applied to the presaturated area, it effectively has received a 180° pulse, and therefore it has no component of transverse magnetization and produces no signal. Consider the sagittal image of the pelvis in Figure 8–17A. Considerable motion artifact

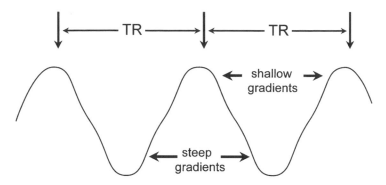

Figure 8–15. Steep phase-encoding gradients are used during end expiration, since there will be little motion to cause artifacts.

is superimposed over an enlarged, myomatous uterus, obscuring detail. If a saturation pulse is applied anterior to the anterior pelvic wall, signal from motion anterior to the saturation pulse is eliminated and there is minimal respiratory artifact in Figure 8–17B. Notice the decreased signal in the subcutaneous fat (arrow), an area that was included in the saturation pulse volume.

Saturation pulses can also be applied in order to eliminate signal from either protons in water or protons in fat. The chemical environments of the protons in water and those in fat are slightly different and, therefore, the precessional frequencies of the two different types of protons are slightly different. The difference depends upon the field strength of the magnet: the higher the field strength, the greater the difference. At 1.5 T, the precessional frequency of protons in fat is 220 Hz less than those in water. Since the precessional frequency is 63 MHz, or 63,000,000 Hz, the difference between fat and water is less than 0.00035%, or about 3 parts per million.

Fat saturation techniques effectively get rid of the fat signal from an image. First, the 90° presaturation pulse of exactly the fat precessional frequency is applied to the entire volume being imaged. Then when the 90° excitation pulse is applied to each slice, the fat protons are effectively flipped to 180°, and again they have no transverse magnetization component and produce no signal. Only the water protons are then capable of producing a signal (Figure 8–18).

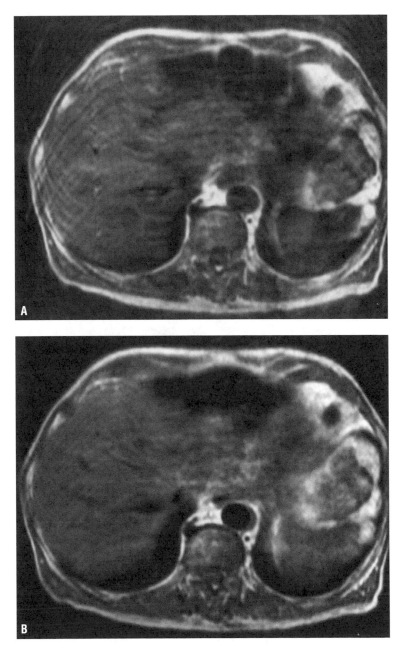

Figure 8–16. (A) Axial image through the liver of an unsteady 89-year-old man shows marked respiratory artifact. (B) Respiratory compensation techniques were applied, and although some artifact remains, there has been a significant improvement in image quality.

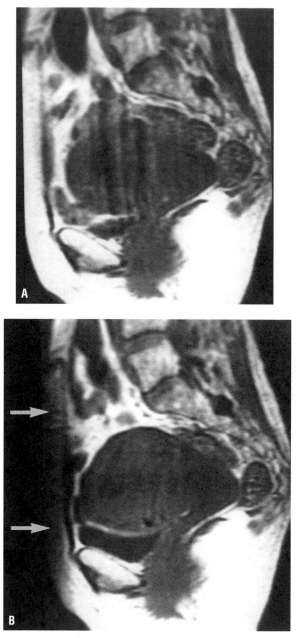

Figure 8–17. (A) Sagittal image of the pelvis with an enlarged myomatous uterus. Respiratory motion artifacts decrease the resolution of the image. (B) The same image as in A, but a presaturation pulse has been placed just on the anterior abdominal wall (arrows), significantly increasing resolution.

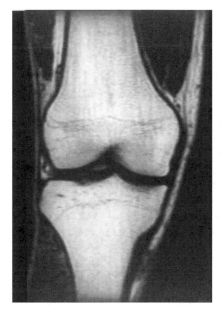 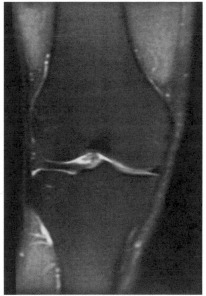

Figure 8–18. In this coronal image of the knee, water-saturation pulses have been applied. The muscle, which contains a large amount of water, is much darker than it normally would be on a T1-weighted image. The subcutaneous fat and fat within the marrow cavity remain bright.

Figure 8–19. This image is anatomically identical to that of Figure 8–18, except that fat- (rather than water-) saturation pulses have been applied. Subcutaneous fat and fat in the marrow cavity have been decreased (suppressed) while the water in the muscles makes them appear relatively bright.

Water saturation techniques are identical, except that the presaturation pulse that is applied is exactly the precessional frequency of the water protons. Then, during the normal imaging process, the water protons do not give a signal and the only signal available is from the fat protons (Figure 8–19). Fat saturation techniques are more commonly utilized than water saturation. Evaluating fatty infiltration of the liver is the only common use for water saturation procedures. Fat saturation is used to distinguish fatty, necrotic, and hemorrhagic components of tumors, and in pre- and postcontrast studies in the evaluation of osteomyelitis, where the bright fat signal in the bone marrow may mask the enhancement of the gadolinium.

CONTRAST AGENTS

A **contrast agent** can be defined as a material that changes the appearance of certain tissues. Contrast agents can be administered orally or intravenously. During CT examinations, both oral and intravenous (and sometimes rectal) contrast are employed. In MR imaging, it is the signal intensity that is altered by the introduction of different materials. These materials can either change the distribution of protons or alter the T1 and T2 relaxation times. Air is one example of a contrast agent that can be used to alter the proton distribution. The concentration of protons in air is extremely low and will give no signal. Air in the lumen of the stomach or bowel will therefore appear black on MR images. Although air is not used routinely, the introduction of air into the gastrointestinal tract can sometimes allow separation of normal and abnormal structures.

The majority of MR contrast materials being investigated involve paramagnetic or ferromagnetic materials, which change the signal intensities of the tissues being investigated. Paramagnetic substances decrease the T1 relaxation times of tissues that they infiltrate, thereby increasing signal from the affected regions and making them appear brighter on T1-weighted images. This brightening of the tissues by administering contrast material is called **contrast enhancement**. The FDA has approved only one element for clinical use as a magnetic contrast agent: the paramagnetic element gadolinium. **Gadolinium** is a rare element, which has seven unpaired electrons when combined in compounds, making it highly paramagnetic. As a pure element it is toxic and can cause serious medical problems, but when tightly bound to a ligand such as DTPA, or HP-DO3A, it can safely be injected intravenously. It is excreted by the kidneys and has an effective half-life of approximately 20 minutes. After injection, it rapidly enters tissues that have a blood supply and helps to identify distinguish tumors from areas of edema, as well as detect many tumors that may not be easily seen by noncontrast studies (Figure 8–20). It is both useful and necessary in the evaluation of the postoperative lumbar spine, where it can be used to differentiate recurrent disk herniations from scar tissue (Figure 8–21). Since many tumors as well as cysts become bright on

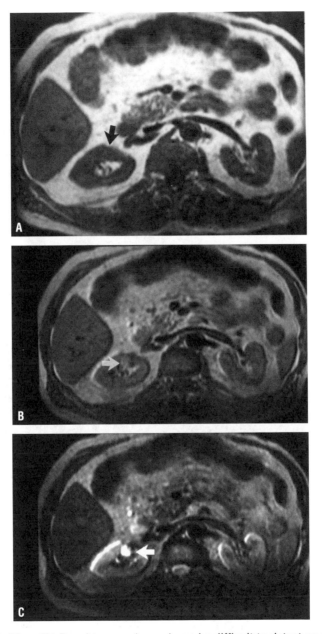

Figure 8–20. (A) Renal tumors (arrow) can be difficult to detect on this spin-echo image. (B) After the administration of gadolinium-DTPA, the increased vascularity of the tumor makes it stand out due to its brighter signal. (C) On this T2-weighted image the tumor is indistinguishable from a renal cyst (see also Figure 8-22).

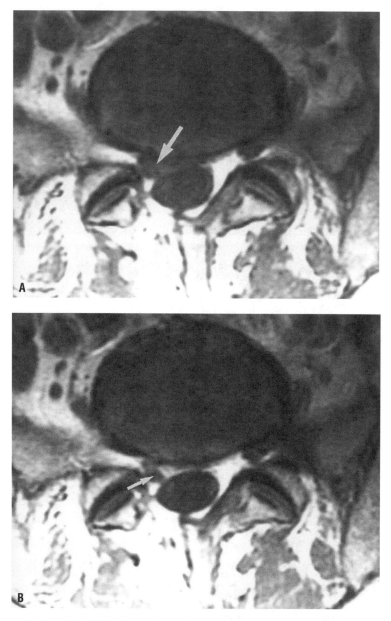

Figure 8–21.   (A) Obliquely sectioned image through an intervertebral disk in a patient who was previously operated upon for a herniated disk. This image shows a region of decreased signal (arrow) that could represent either a recurrent disk herniation or scar tissue. (B) After the administration of gadolinium-DTPA, the region becomes bright due to the vascularity of the scar tissue. Arrow points to nerve root.

the T2-weighted images, injection of gadolinium-DTPA can be effective in determining whether a lesion is a cyst or a solid, vascular mass (Figure 8–22).

Gadolinium-DTPA is usually used with T1-weighted images. The plane (or planes) that best delineate the area being investigated are scanned before injection to provide a precontrast image. The patient should be cautioned not to move during the injection so that the same positioning parameters can be used for the postcontrast images. This consistency allows a direct comparison of the pre- and postinjection images in order to determine if there was enhancement by the lesion. Imaging should be performed right after injection. Since fat is bright on the T1-weighted images, it may obscure areas becoming bright due to contrast material. For this reason, some types of pathology are imaged using fat-suppression techniques, as mentioned before.

Ferromagnetic materials decrease the T2-relaxation times of tissues, causing a decrease in signal. This T2 effect is, not surprisingly, most apparent on T2-weighted images. Ferromagnetic contrast agents have been used in experimental studies to decrease signal from normal liver and permit abnormal lesions to be better seen, and also as oral contrast to delineate the gastrointestinal tract. Oral contrast material is not often used in clinical studies, however.

FLOW COMPENSATION

Flow compensation, also called gradient moment nulling or gradient moment rephasing, is utilized to eliminate ghosting artifact from flowing blood or CSF pulsations (Figure 8–23). Protons that are moving through applied magnetic gradients will acquire phase shifts relative to stationary protons. This phase shift results in a ghosting artifact in the phase-encoding gradient, equal to the width of the blood vessel.

Flow compensation will apply compensating gradients that will correct for the acquired phase shifts, so that there will be no difference in phase between moving blood or CSF and nonmoving tissues at the echo time, TE, the time at which the echo is acquired. Since this process requires using additional

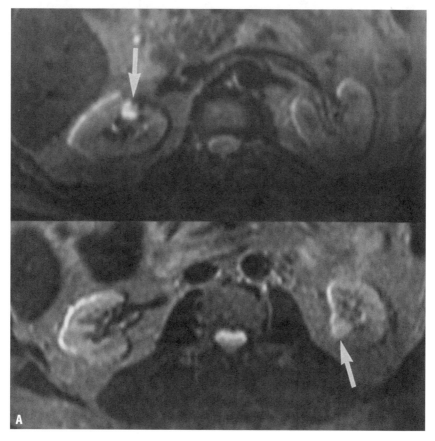

Figure 8–22. (A) On T-2 weighted images both tumor (arrow, top image) and cyst (arrow, bottom image) become bright.

compensating gradients, it takes more time before the data acquisition can begin, so that the minimum TE is increased and fewer slices can be obtained for a given sequence. The technique is most effective for constant flow velocities and is not as effective with rapid, turbulent, or pulsatile flow. It is also very effective in minimizing artifact when scanning after the intravenous injection of gadolinium base contrast. Gradient moment nulling increases signal from blood and is most often used in T2-weighted or gradient-echo sequences, where fluid is normally

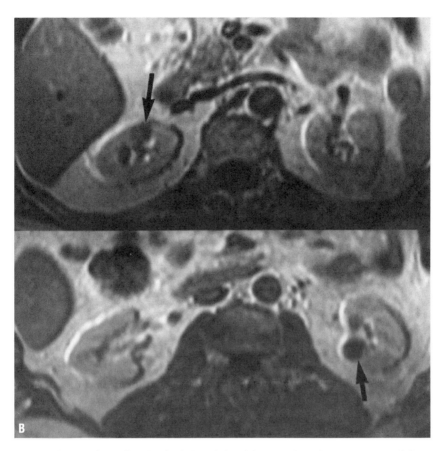

Figure 8–22. *(cont.)* (B) On T1-weighted image after the intravenous injection of gadolinium-DTPA there is some enhancement by the tumor (arrow, top image) because it has a blood supply, but the cyst (arrow, bottom image) remains very dark, because it has no blood supply.

bright (Figure 8–24). There is a displacement of signal when flow compensation is used with very long echo times and if the blood vessel is slightly oblique to the imaging plane. What this amounts to is that the blood vessel is "mismapped"; that is, it appears in the wrong place in the scan. This artifact must be kept in mind when using this technique with long echo sequences.

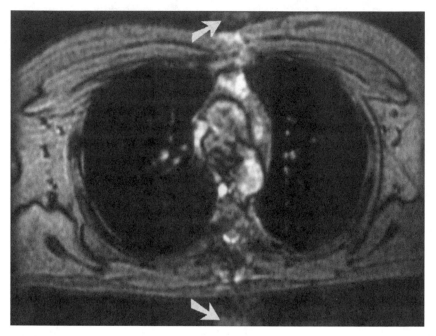

Figure 8–23. A flow artifact (arrows) can be observed propagating through this image in the phase-encoding direction, causing a blurring of mediastinal structures in this gradient-echo image at the level just below the aortic arch.

PHASE, FREQUENCY, AND FIELD OF VIEW

While the field of view (FOV) is regarded as a routine imaging parameter, the direction of the phase- and frequency-encoding gradients are not usually considered in this category. Proper selection of the phase- and frequency-encoding directions, along with an appropriate FOV, can become invaluable imaging tools to identify and eliminate artifacts and to significantly decrease imaging time as well. The effect of changing FOVs as a single variable has been discussed in the previous chapter.

As discussed earlier, gradients can be applied in the three orthogonal directions: the z-axis gradient is the slice-selection gradient; the x-axis gradient is the frequency-encoding gradient; the y-axis gradient is the phase-encoding gradient. By convention, in the sagittal plane the phase-encoding direction is anterior-posterior and the frequency-encoding direction is superior-anterior; in the axial plane the phase-encoding direction is anterior-posterior

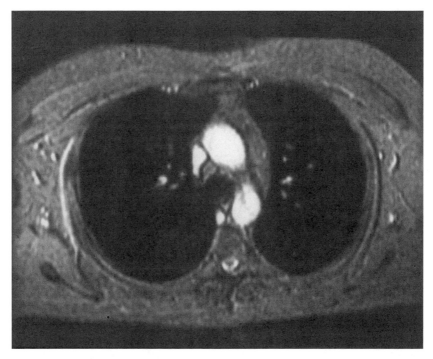

Figure 8–24.   By applying flow compensation to the sequence used to obtain Figure 8–23, the resulting artifact and decreased resolution are minimized. Note that the signal of flowing blood is brighter with flow compensation than without it.

and the frequency-encoding direction is left-right (reversed for head coil); in the coronal plane the phase-encoding direction is left-right and the frequency-encoding direction is superior-anterior. These are conventions only and can easily be switched with current software, if necessary.

Motion artifacts (Chapter 10) are propagated in the direction of the phase-encoding gradient. As illustrated in Figure 8–12, switching the phase and frequency directions will switch the direction of the transmission of the motion-induced signal and may aid in the interpretation of the image. Utilizing the directions of the phase- and frequency-encoding gradients together with the FOV can aid in decreasing image time without any loss of resolution. This is, obviously, a great help in working with anxious patients and also useful when working with a tightly packed schedule.

Observing images, it is apparent that in some cases, large portions of the imaged volume contain empty space. If data acquisition of the empty area can be eliminated, the total scanning time will be shortened. This can be accomplished by pruning the extremes of the phase-encoding gradient. Choices now available permit the operator to choose either ¾ FOV or ½ FOV options. If the ¾ FOV option is chosen, data from the extreme one-eighth of each end of the phase-encoding axis is not collected (Figure 8–25A). This option can be chosen only if there is no

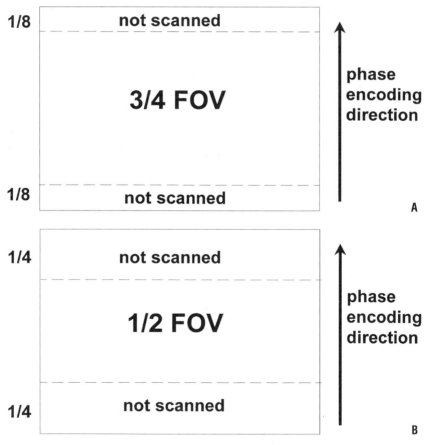

Figure 8–25.   (A) Using a ¾ FOV, one-quarter of the field of view is not scanned—half (one-eighth) on one edge of the phase-encoding direction and half (one-eighth) on the opposite edge. (B) Using a ½ FOV, one-half of the field of view is not scanned—half (one-fourth) on one edge of the phase-encoding direction and half (one-fourth) on the opposite edge.

anatomy in the region being cut away. This will cut down the imaging time by 25%, which is significant on a long acquisition sequence. Similarly, the ½ FOV option will cut out the extreme one-quarter of the volume at each end of the phase-encoding direction and will decrease imaging time by one-half (Figure 8–25B). If there is any anatomy in the "pruned" region, a wrap-around artifact will ensue (Figure 8–26), so the operator must be

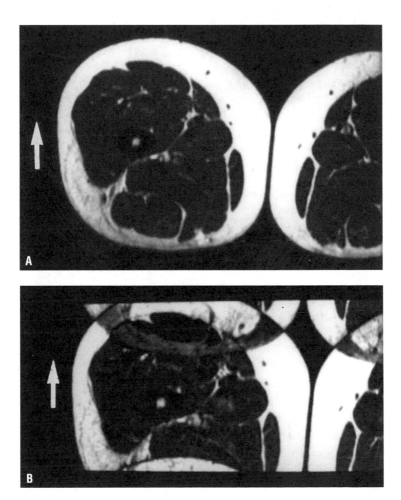

Figure 8–26.   (A) Use of a ¾ FOV decreased imaging time of this thigh by 25%, since the area above and below the legs (containing just air) did not have to be scanned. (B) Use of a ½ FOV decreased imaging time by 50%, but the resulting field of view was too small, leaving tissue in the adjacent nonsampled area, resulting in a wrap-around artifact.

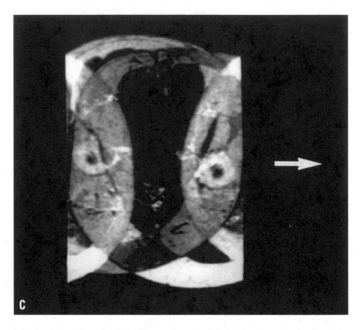

Figure 8–26. *(cont.)*   (C) Utilizing a fractional FOV when phase and frequency have been switched decreases the desired field of view in the wrong direction and results in a severe wrap-around artifact. (Arrows indicate direction of the phase-encoding gradient.)

certain that the proper directions are chosen for both phase- and frequency-encoding gradients. For example, an axial section of the abdomen approximates an oval with the major axis running left to right (Figure 8–27). The anterior and posterior aspect of the image contain space, so a fractional field of view can be used if the phase-encoding direction runs anterior-posterior. An axial image of the head approximates an oval with the major axis running anterior to posterior. The left and right aspects of the image contain space, so a fractional field of view can be used if the phase-encoding direction runs left to right (Figure 8–28). In situations where the image is not centered within the magnet, an offset is usually necessary in order to use this technique (Figure 8–29). Proper application of this procedure can save a considerable amount of time without loss of image resolution.

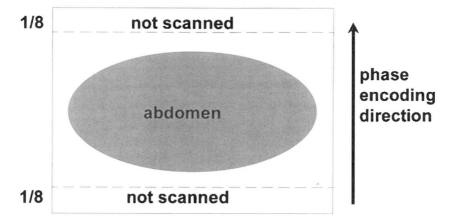

Figure 8–27.   Approximating an axial image of an abdomen by an oval, use of the fractional FOVs will decrease scanning time.

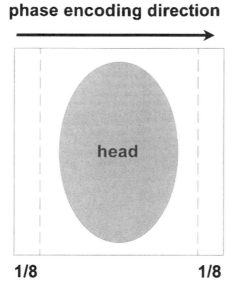

Figure 8–28.   Approximating an axial image of a head by an oval, use of the fractional FOVs will decrease scanning. The nonscanned area is always in the direction of the phase-encoding gradient.

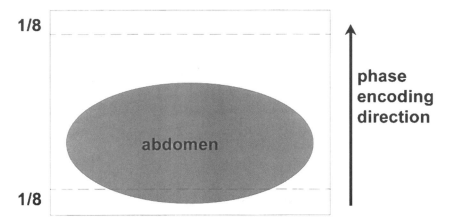

Figure 8–29.   If the portion of the anatomy is not centered within the magnet, an offset must be applied before a fractional FOV can be used; otherwise part of the anatomy will not be imaged and will cause a wrap-around artifact.

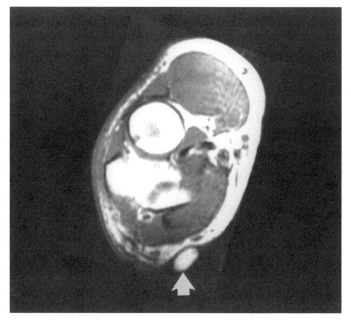

Figure 8–30.   Palpable elbow mass, with area of mass marked with oil capsule (arrow) taped directly over it.

Patients will often be sent for a scan with a vague diagnosis of pain or of a palpable "mass." Imaging the proper area can sometimes be a problem, since specific regions are not provided. In these instances the easiest way to be sure that the area of interest is being imaged is to tape an oil capsule over the area of localized pain or of the palpated mass (Figure 8–30). Subcutaneous lipomas are a very common medical finding and will blend in to the subcutaneous fat, where it will not be distinctive on MRI. On an unmarked study it cannot be established that the proper area was scanned. If the area is marked in some way, it can easily be established that the region was well covered by the MRI examination.

POINTS TO PONDER

- Physiologic motion is an inherent cause of image degradation when scanning the chest, abdomen, and pelvis.

- ECG gating can be used in the chest to decrease artifact caused by cardiac pulsation.

- ECG gating will trigger or begin the TR interval on the R wave of the tracing.

- The TR can be increased when using ECG-gating techniques by programming the system to trigger on every second, third, or fourth R wave.

- The trigger window is a period of dead time at the end of the ECG cycle during which no data is acquired.

- The trigger delay is a period of dead time at the beginning of the cycle, when motion is at a maximum.

- Peripheral gating is useful in imaging patients with cardiac arrhythmias.

- CINE images are rapidly acquired images that cover different phases of the cardiac cycle. When these images are played back rapidly, cardiac motion can be assessed.

POINTS TO PONDER   *(continued)*

- Respiratory motion artifact can be minimized by several methods: breath-holding techniques, true respiratory gating, respiratory compensation, and saturation pulses.

- Saturation techniques involve placing a 90° pulse over the desired area before applying the excitation pulse.

- The effect of the saturation pulse is to eliminate any contribution from the area covered by the saturation pulse.

- Signal from fat and water can also be eliminated with saturation pulses.

- Paramagnetic contrast agents decrease effective T1 values of tissues, causing them to appear brighter on T1-weighted images.

- Gadolinium compounds are the only intravenous contrast agents currently approved by the FDA.

- Flow compensation eliminates ghosting artifact from flowing blood.

CHAPTER NINE

BIOLOGICAL EFFECTS AND SAFETY PRECAUTIONS IN MAGNETIC FIELDS

Safety is a prime consideration when any new medical procedure is introduced. Magnetic resonance imaging does not use ionizing radiation, has not been shown to have any harmful effects on patients or operators, and has been subjected to the most intense investigation of intrinsic safety of any medical modalities. Even so, MRI has not been given unqualified approval by the U.S. Food and Drug Administration (FDA). Although the imaging procedure itself has been deemed safe for routine imaging insofar as the lack of ionizing radiation, the lack of harmful effects of exposure to the magnetic fields and noninvasiveness, there are many considerations that the responsible technologist and physician must be aware of. New pulse sequences, hardware, and techniques also must be continually retested when they are introduced.

Because of problems encountered in the past, any new technology or drug is subjected to rigorous testing procedures before it may be used by or for the general public. Federal testing standards have been established because of multiple instances in which insufficient knowledge about a particular procedure has or could have led to tragic consequences. Radioactive substances, discovered in the late nineteenth century, fascinated the greatest scientific minds of the day, but a lack of information about the biological side-effects of radiation led to the deaths of many of these scientists from radiation-induced cancer. Marie and Pierre Curie were awarded the Nobel Prize for the discovery of and subsequent research with radioactive elements. During World War I, Marie devoted her time to researching the medical uses of X-rays. Although Pierre died after being hit by a truck in 1896, Marie's death from leukemia is attributed to the cumulative effects of a lifetime of overexposure to radiation. The development of fluoroscopy as a diagnostic tool led to its commercial application in the 1940s; it was used as a routine screening procedure in shoe stores to determine correctness of fit of customers' shoes. Both the operator and the customer received large doses of radiation. Fortunately this practice was stopped once the potential hazards of this unnecessary radiation were understood.

The drug thalidomide is an important agent in combatting host-versus-graft disease in patients who have received bone-marrow transplants, an effective drug against leprosy, and a possible agent against rheumatoid arthritis. In the 1960s, however, it was marketed as a remedy for relief of the nausea and vomiting referred to as "morning sickness" during pregnancy. Unfortunately, this was before there had been sufficient research into its effects on the fetus. The resulting birth defects, most commonly to arms and legs, are well documented. For these and many similar cases, the FDA now has the responsibility of approving all new drugs and equipment before they can be utilized, in order to safeguard the public.

Of all of the diagnostic modalities in use today, magnetic resonance imaging has without doubt been submitted to the most exhaustive and extensive testing ever performed. Since it was first applied to imaging by Dr. Paul Lauterbur in 1971, scientists have performed experimentation of almost every conceivable type in order to assure its safety, both long and short term, in general use. Safety is a multifaceted concern, and with MRI, it must be assured for such diverse issues as the effects of both static and changing magnetic fields on the body, on miscellaneous objects in the magnet room, and on surgically implanted devices; the effects on pregnant women and on the fetuses that they carry; the effects of radiofrequencies used during the procedure; and the potential consequences of a malfunction in the equipment.

It is important to realize that safety is relative. Materials that are considered totally safe can become dangerous in certain circumstances. Pure water, when spilled on a tile floor, can become a potential source of head trauma, should someone slip on it. A needle and thread can be used by a skilled surgeon to close an operative site, or to create a fancy gown when used by a seamstress, but they are a source of likely peril in the hands of a child. Relative safety is a most important concept in magnetic resonance imaging. "Familiarity breeds contempt," goes the old adage, and this can be very true in MRI, where the potential for problems must always be kept in mind. In this chapter on safety, we want to discuss the various aspects relating to the care and security of both patients and technical personnel working in magnetic fields.

MAGNETIC FIELDS, GRADIENTS, AND RADIOFREQUENCY

Stationary magnetic fields of up to 2.0 T are considered safe to humans and without hazardous or unpleasant side effects. Although early experiments suggested potential problems, other scientists were unable to reproduce this initial work. It is now accepted that there is no evidence of biological risk to humans or their DNA for exposure to static magnetic fields below 2.0 T. High magnetic fields are relatively common in many frequently encountered situations: stereo speakers can generate fields of over 500 G; small electric motors can generate fields of several hundred gauss; a seat over a transformer on a subway car is exposed to a field of about 300 G; the magnetic field of the center of an atom has been estimated to be over 300,000 G.

Higher field strengths, however, have not been "cleared" of potential effects. Several 4.0-T MRI systems are currently operational and, while they are not FDA-approved, they are scanning patients on a research basis. As far back as 1983, reports of flashes of light appearing before a person's eyes were observed for patients moving in high magnetic fields. These visual effects are called magnetophosphenes. They are thought to be caused either by rapidly changing high magnetic fields, or by motion within a magnetic field. A level of 4.0 T appears high enough to cause this phenomenon. Additional effects experienced at static 4.0 T, but not at 2.0 T, include vertigo, dizziness, and headaches. These effects are reproducible and are felt by patients in static magnetic fields, although experts believe that they are the result of eye and/or head movement within the static field, which produces the effect of a rapidly changing system.

Magnetic gradients produce rapidly changing magnetic fields during the scanning process. As has been discussed, scan location, slice thickness, pulse thickness, field of view, and pixel size are some of the many variables that are controlled by applying magnetic gradients during the imaging process. All biological effects attributed to changing magnetic fields are due to the fact that changing magnetic fields are able to produce small electrical currents in biological systems. The higher the field strength, the more intense the induced current. The more rapidly the gradients are changing and the larger the gradient, the more likely a current is to be induced in tissue. Magnetophosphenes, for example, are thought to be the result of induced currents in the optic nerve, and they have even been experienced by blind patients.

MRI systems currently in clinical use can induce currents in tissue; however, they are not high enough to cause biological effects. As summarized by Shellock and Kanal,[1] current densities produced by 1.5-T systems (without echo-planar capabilities) are of the order of 3 μA/cm^2. Current densities of 15 to 100 μA/cm^2 are needed to produce the contraction of skeletal muscle. Seizures can conceivably be caused by induced currents, but the threshold is approximately one million times higher than can be produced with imaging equipment. Patients suffer no cardiac effects below 2.0 T, but several workers utilizing echo-planar imaging have reported palpitations in patients.

Induced currents can be easily produced in wires by changing magnetic fields. For this reason patients with pacemakers or those who have pacing wires in their chests cannot have an MR examination. Currents will be produced in the wire even at low field strengths, and will stimulate the cardiac muscles to contract, with the potentially disastrous prospect of putting the patient into ventricular fibrillation. While static fields at and below 2.0 T do not produce any unhealthy biological effects, high gradient fields that are rapidly changing, such as those used in echo-planar imaging, have the potential to bring on unwanted results.

MR imaging does not use harmful ionizing radiation (such as X-rays or gamma rays), which can destroy cells and produce changes in DNA, but it does use radiofrequency radiation. As discussed in Chapter 3, rf waves are a low-energy form of electromagnetic radiation that is usually considered harmless. As used in MRI, there is a concern about how much radiation is employed during the study. Much of the rf energy enters the body: some of it excites the protons and is re-emitted; some of it simply stays in the body tissues, where it is quickly converted into heat energy. The concern is over how much heat energy is deposited in the tissues. If heat energy is added to any object, it will heat up and then radiate heat energy as it cools down to its original temperature. With the appearance of high-field MRI units in the mid-1980s, the FDA expressed a genuine concern that body temperatures might be elevated to too high a level during prolonged examinations. Imaging times, number of slices, and total number of sequences were severely limited at first, so that the specific absorption rate (SAR)—the rate at which energy is absorbed by tissue—fell within certain specified limits. Weight was the major factor in determining the number of images permitted during an examination: the heavier the patient, the fewer the number of slices allowed. The reasoning was that the heavier the patient, the more likely he or she was to have excess subcutaneous fat. Since fat is an excellent insulator, heat deposited within the body would not be lost as easily as it would be in a thin person. Much detailed experimentation and many years of clinical experience showed that the precautions were not necessary, as even during very long examinations, relatively little change in body temperature was ever noted, usually between 0.10°F and 1°F. Although tissue heating is no longer an issue at 1.5 T, significantly more heat is deposited in tissues at 4 T, and these research magnets are being closely monitored so that SAR limits are not exceeded.

PREGNANCY

For new procedures and medications, most concern is expressed for the safety of the pregnant patient. The question of whether to permit pregnant patients to be scanned has been controversial because of possible adverse effects to the mother and fetus resulting from exposure to the magnetic fields, both static and changing, and to rf electromagnetic fields. Although most data substantiate the position that MR imaging is safe for both the mother and fetus, there is some questionable but still conflicting data on cell cultures and lower forms of animal life, especially in the very early stages of embryogenesis. Because of these controversies, MR imaging of the pregnant patient has not yet been approved by the FDA, however, neither has it been disapproved by them.

In practice, there are no set policies among MR centers. Some centers will not perform the procedure on pregnant patients at all,[2] while others will perform it at any point during the pregnancy and still others will perform it only after the first trimester. The official policy stated by the Safety Committee of the Society for Magnetic Resonance Imaging reads:

> MR imaging may be used in pregnant women if other non-ionizing forms of diagnostic imaging are inadequate or if the examination provides important information that would otherwise require exposure to ionizing radiation (e.g., fluoroscopy, CT, etc.). It is recommended that pregnant patients be informed that, to date, there has been no indication that the use of clinical MR imaging during pregnancy has produced deleterious effects. However, as noted by the FDA, the safety of MR imaging during pregnancy has not been proved.[3]

This is essentially the procedure that we follow at The New York Hospital–Cornell University Medical Center. While we prefer to wait until the end of the first trimester, unless the working diagnosis is life-threatening or disabling (such as cord compression), we will image pregnant patients. The patient is informed by a physician, technologist, or nurse that although no harmful effects have been demonstrated to either the mother or fetus, the procedure has not been approved by the FDA for pregnant patients. To ensure that the patient has been properly advised, she is asked to sign an appropriate informed-consent document.

No deleterious effects of static MR fields have been demonstrated for pregnant MR technologists, physicians, and nurses. For these workers, two different situations must be considered: entering the room with a static magnetic field; and remaining in the room during the study, which involves exposure to gradient magnetic fields and rf electromagnetic fields. While the exposure to a patient is a single short-term effect, for an MR worker, continued exposure would be a chronic situation.

A study of over 1,900 female MR technologists who reported over 1,400 pregnancies did not demonstrate any differences from the same group of employees before they became MR workers.[4] Categories such as early delivery, low birth weight, gender, infertility, menstrual regularity, and miscarriages were compared and showed no significant differences. In their text on bioeffects and safety of MR procedures, Shellock and Kanal state that data obtained is reassuring that there are no harmful effects to the pregnant MR worker or her fetus when working in a static magnetic field, and they recommend that pregnant health care workers should continue to perform MR procedures, entering the magnet room and attending to the patient. However, they do suggest that such workers do not remain in the room while the actual scanning is being performed.[5]

This difference in recommendation is due to the differences in what is occurring during the data acquisition as opposed to in between scans. During idle periods when no scanning is being performed, the only effect to be concerned with is the static magnetic field. Throughout the scanning procedure, gradients are changing and rf energy is being released. Accepting the old adage "discretion is the better part of valor," it is felt that even though the risks are minimal, if they exist at all, it is better for a pregnant nurse, technologist, or physician to remain outside of the scanning room while scans are being performed.

SOUND

Much of this chapter has been devoted to the effects of gradients. The gradients are also responsible for the loud knocking or banging noises associated with MR scanning. The gradient coils are embedded in solid material around the bore of the magnet. When a current is introduced into a gradient coil, it produces a large force, which tends to try to make the coil move. This results in the very loud noise with each application of a gradient pulse.

The loudness of a noise is measured in decibels. Decibels are defined by a logarithmic scale, which means that an increase of one decibel indicates that the noise level has increased ten times. Table 9–1 lists decibel levels for several familiar sources of noise. The decibel level of noise within the magnet (the noise that a patient would hear) varies from about 83 to 95 and depends upon the pulse sequence used. Noise levels, which were already loud with earlier techniques, have significantly

TABLE 9-1. DECIBEL LEVELS OF NOISE FROM COMMON SOURCES

Decibels	Source of Noise
0	Softest audible sound
10	Whisper
20	Rustling of leaves
30	A quiet street in the evening
40	Normal conversation
50	Riding in an automobile
70	Average big city street noises
75	Traffic in a busy city intersection
90	20 feet from an elevated city train
83–95	**Various MRI pulse sequences**
100	Speeding express train
100	35 feet from a riveter
110	10 feet from a jack hammer
120	Very nearby thunder
130	Rock concert
130	Working in a boiler factory

increased with the introduction of new fast spin-echo sequences, during which gradient changes are larger and are made much more rapidly. This noise affects individuals in very different ways, but increased anxiety, headaches, and temporary hearing loss are common complaints. One study reported a temporary hearing loss in 43% of all patients scanned without ear protection.[6] For these reasons, earplugs should be given to all patients. Patients who refuse earplugs, claiming that they have not had a problem in previous examinations, should nevertheless be encouraged to use them, since they may not have been exposed to the higher decibel level with the new pulse sequences. Music systems, employing headphones that decrease the gradient knocking while piping in music, offer the additional advantage of decreasing patient anxiety as they listen to music that they find pleasing. Antinoise systems, which can profoundly minimize noise, have also been proposed.[7] These procedures use a computer analysis of the actual MR noise that is produced and generate a noise identical to it, but exactly opposite in phase, so that the combination of the two will cancel out.

There are federal guidelines for maximum noise levels to which every manufacturer is required to adhere. This noise level is based upon a long-term (chronic) exposure to noise. Table 9–2 lists the limits imposed on the maximum amount of noise to

TABLE 9-2. LENGTH OF PERMITTED OCCUPATIONAL EXPOSURE AT DIFFERENT ACOUSTIC LEVELS

Noise Level (Decibels)	Maximum Hours Allowed per Day
90	8.00
92	6.00
95	4.00
97	3.00
100	1.50
102	1.00
105	0.50
115	0.25

Source: Federal guidelines adapted from Shellock FG and Kanal E: *Magnetic Resonance: Bioeffects, Safety, and Patient Management.* New York: Raven Press; 1994: 51.

which a worker can be exposed for a given amount of time in the work area. Levels for chronic exposure are of concern to MR technologists who are constantly working in a noisy environment. Since the patient is exposed for only a short time, the noise produced during the examination is considerably below a level of concern for any permanent auditory damage.

Related to potential problems associated with the sound made by the imaging system are patients wearing hearing aids. This is often a fact that patients are reluctant to disclose; this question must be asked by the technologist, and should be included in the patient questionnaire. *All hearing aids must be removed before a patient is scanned.* Two different issues are involved here. First, the strong magnetic field will very often ruin the device, making it inoperable and therefore worthless. Second, if the unit is not rendered ineffective, it will serve to amplify the sound heard by the patient in the magnet, increasing the level of noise discomfort substantially.

CONTRAST AGENTS

As with all medications, the gadolinium-based contrast agents currently approved for use in MR imaging were subjected to exhaustive testing before being pronounced safe for general use. Gadolinium is a paramagnetic substance that becomes very bright on T1-weighted images; it is very useful as an MR contrast agent. The free gadolinium ion, however, is quite toxic, affecting the brain and causing an irreversible pseudo-Parkinson's condition. The free ion remains in the system for a relatively long time, as the kidneys eliminate it only slowly. By combining the ion with chelating agents that are very tightly bound to the gadolinium ion, the characteristics are quite drastically changed.

Three MR contrast agents are currently approved by the FDA: Magnevist (Gd-DTPA, gadolinium diethylenetriamine pentaacetic acid, Berlex Laboratories), in which the gadolinium ion is bound to the DTPA chelate, resulting in an ionic contrast material; Omniscan (Gd-DTPA-BMA, gadolinium diethylenetriamine pentaacetic acid bismethylamide, Sanofi-Winthrop Pharmaceuticals), a non-ionic molecule; and ProHance

(Gd-DO3A, gadoteridol, Squibb Diagnostics), another non-ionic molecule in which a chelate is combined with gadolinium. Each of these chelating agents is very tightly bound to the gadolinium ion in a nontoxic compound that is cleared from the body relatively quickly, with half-lives of less than two hours. The difference between ionic and non-ionic contrast is negligible from a safety point of view (as opposed to the situation with CT contrast), since the amount of material injected is small and the differences in osmotic loads are insignificant.

Adverse reactions are minor and have a reported incidence of 2 to 4%. Reactions most often observed include nausea, headaches, hives, and irritation from extravasation into the subcutaneous tissues during injection. Our experience has been that nausea and headaches, although observed infrequently, are almost always associated with a very rapid injection. We have observed hives in a few patients who have had a history of severe allergies. Incidents of anaphylactoid reactions are rare, but have been reported.

Even though gadolinium contrast agents are considered safe, they are not indicated for all patients. There is concern that diminished clearance of contrast in patients in renal failure or with severely diminished renal function may result in the chelated complex remaining in the body for a long enough period of time to release free gadolinium ion, which is toxic. In these patients, contrast should be used only when absolutely necessary, and even then it appears prudent to use as low a dose as possible. In vitro experiments have demonstrated that gadolinium contrast added to blood of patients with sickle cell anemia causes the sickled red blood cells to align themselves perpendicular to an applied magnetic field. This could conceivably cause a blood clot in vivo; however, there have been no reports of any complications to sickle cell patients who have received gadolinium contrast.

Although no conclusive studies have yet been published, our approach is to withhold contrast from pregnant females. The gadolinium chelates have been shown to cross the placental barrier quickly. They would then enter the fetal bloodstream, be filtered by the fetal kidneys, and be excreted into the amniotic fluid. A cycle would then be established in which the fetus would swallow the amniotic fluid, it would enter the blood-stream, be filtered by the kidneys into the amniotic fluid, and be swallowed again. The possibility exists that the chelate would remain in the fetal circulation for a sufficiently long time for it to produce some free gadolinium ion. Until there are sufficient studies to prove the safety of gadolinium to the fetus, we urge a conservative approach.

Contrast has also been shown to be excreted with human breast milk in nursing mothers for almost 36 hours. Nursing mothers should therefore be told in advance of receiving the contrast injection that it would be best if they refrain from nursing for 48 hours. This is a conservative approach, since gadolinium contrast is only very slightly absorbed through the gastrointestinal tract.

MAGNETIC ATTRACTION

It has already been stated that magnetic fields will not produce any harmful biological effects. Magnetic attraction, however, can sometimes lead to a fatal attraction under certain circumstances. One such situation is the so-called **missile effect**. Magnetic fields will attract magnetic material, and strong magnetic fields will attract magnetic material with an appreciable force. If a patient is lying within the bore of the magnet and someone enters the magnet room with something that can be attracted by the magnetic field (pen, keys, paper clips, hair pins, stethoscope, scalpel, etc.), it can easily be pulled out of a pocket and fly through the air towards the center of the magnet as if it were a missile. Even a paper clip can be dangerous if it attains a velocity of 30 miles per hour, which is possible at 1.5 T. A sharp object or a large object fly-ing into the bore of the magnet could easily strike a patient, with potentially disastrous consequences. Care must be taken to ensure that no one enters the scanning room with loose metallic objects in their pockets. Anyone working in the area regularly will soon get used to checking for metallic objects. The major prob-lems usually occur when transient personnel come in. This group may include the patient's physician, family members, medical students, and the like. Technologists and physicians working in MRI units must constantly be on the alert that someone may bring a potentially dangerous item into the room. Signs should be posted at the entrance, and entering personnel should always be questioned and reminded to leave metallic objects outside. Even seemingly innocuous objects can sometimes cause problems. The recently replaced New York City subway tokens (still used on buses) are made of copper (non-magnetic) but contain a central core of highly magnetic stainless steel. These tokens are frequently pulled out of patients' pockets as they are lying on the table; if they lodge under the patient table, they are found only after a search for unexplained metallic artifacts.

In addition to warning against bringing metallic objects into the scanning room, everyone entering should be reminded that magnetic fields can also have negative effects on other items. The magnetic strips on credit and bank cards will be erased by the field and thus will no longer be able to be "read" by any electronic device. These cards can still be used in some situations, but they will appear blank to any electronic reader, such as an automated teller machine at a bank, and will have to be replaced. A nondigital watch can have its cog wheels magnetized, rendering it useless for anything except remembering the time when you entered the magnet room. Many jewelers can degauss the watch, but very often the cost is more than the value of the watch. Paging devices (beepers) and other electronic equipment can be permanently ruined by the high magnetic field.

As previously noted (Chapter 5), the FDA guidelines suggest that restricted access be required for all areas where the magnetic field strength is 5 G or greater. While this is not a firm requirement, this guideline is observed in almost all MRI centers, to prevent access to anyone who may be harmed by strong magnetic fields or anyone unfamiliar with the problems associated with magnetic fields.

SURGICALLY IMPLANTED DEVICES

Many metallic objects are placed in the body for a variety of reasons. In view of the preceding discussion, metallic and electronic objects that have been implanted into the body, surgically or otherwise, require careful consideration. For the purposes of this discussion we can consider an apparatus a "device" if it causes something to happen or to move or to keep from moving. "Devices" therefore include pacemakers, which make the heart contract; implanted infusion pumps, which cause medication to enter the bloodstream; magnetic dental implants, which keep dental prostheses in place; cochlear implants, which cause the tympanic membrane to move, improving hearing; and magnetic ocular prostheses, which employ magnetic attraction to keep the prostheses in place. We can consider something an "implement" if it functions solely to replace a bone (hip prosthesis) or has been implanted to surgically aid in healing (aneurysm clip, ventricular shunt, sternal sutures, bypass clips). We consider it a "foreign body" if it has accidentally become lodged within the body (shrapnel, bullet, metallic splinter in the eye).

Any patient with an electronic or magnetic device is not a candidate for an MRI procedure. Patients with pacemakers, neurostimulating devices, and implanted infusion pumps cannot have MR studies and should not even enter the scanning room. The strong magnetic field can cause permanent damage to these devices. As discussed before, the pacing wire in a pacemaker causes an additional problem, since a current is induced in the pacing wire and causes unwanted cardiac contractions. Even patients in whom the pacemaker is known to be nonfunctioning cannot have an MR examination because the pacing wire is still in place and may cause associated problems. Another contraindication to MR imaging is a patient with a cochlear implant. Cochlear implants can employ magnetic or electronic means to improve hearing, and MR studies should never be attempted in these patients. Patients wearing Holter monitors to record cardiac activity cannot be scanned while wearing the recorder, which will be permanently damaged by the magnetic field. Since they must wear the mechanism for 24 hours, the MR examination must be rescheduled for a time when they are not being monitored. Although some devices are expressly manufactured to be MR compatible, definite verification must be made in each case before a patient can be scanned.

Metallic objects will usually cause a metallic artifact on the images (Chapter 10) and may or may not be affected by a magnetic field, although most objects in the body will not be moved when placed in the magnet. A metallic "implement" is usually safe, whether it is magnetic or not, with one major exception—cerebral aneurysm clips. A cerebral aneurysm clip is placed on an aneurysm of a cerebral artery to keep it from a potentially fatal rupture. Although MR systems are not strong enough to significantly move implanted surgical hardware, it had been thought that in the case of cerebral aneurysm clips, only a small torque, or force, would be necessary to rotate the clip a few degrees. This is all that would be necessary to tear the wall of the artery and cause a fatal bleed (Figure 9–1). Patients with cerebral aneurysm clips, therefore, historically have been another group that has been excluded from having MRI examinations.

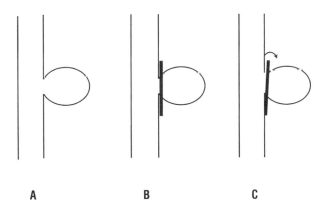

A   B   C

Figure 9–1. A cerebral aneurysm is a ballooning or bulging out of a weakened part of the wall of a cerebral artery (A). The most effective way to repair this defect is to place a cerebral aneurysm clamp over the neck of the aneurysm (B). If this clamp is magnetic, and the patient enters a strong magnetic field, it does not have to move appreciably, but just a slight torque could move it very slightly, causing a tear in the wall of the artery, which could lead to a fatal bleed (C).

During the past ten years, as MRI has evolved as a major imaging modality, most manufacturers of surgical hardware have begun to manufacture nonmagnetic surgical appliances so that they will not interfere with the scan or with a patient's ability to have a scan. Cerebral aneurysm clips have been manufactured from nonmagnetic material in recent years so that patients in whom they have been used would no longer be excluded from having MRI examinations. It cannot be too strongly stressed how important it is to be absolutely certain that the cerebral aneurysm clip of a patient to be scanned is nonmagnetic. A recent report documents the death, from a fatal cerebral hemorrhage, of a patient with a reported aneurysm clip during an MRI study.[8] An autopsy revealed that the clip was actually ferromagnetic.

Most other surgical implements are usually safe for MR imaging, including bypass clips; knee, hip, elbow, and wrist prostheses; sternal sutures; cardiac valves; vascular filters; and ventricular shunts. These implements may produce metallic artifact in the image, but the magnetic field will not harm the patient or damage the object. If there is the slightest doubt, the examination should be rescheduled until the manufacturer and model number of the object are determined and checked out conclusively. Table 9–3 lists implanted objects that eliminate a patient as a candidate for an MRI exam.

"Foreign bodies" are pieces of metal that accidentally enter the body—for example, bullets, shrapnel, pellets (buckshot, BBs, etc.), and slivers of metal in the eye or other part of

TABLE 9-3. PATIENTS EXCLUDED FROM HAVING MRI EXAMINATIONS

Patients with cerebral aneurysm clips[1]
Patients with pacemakers or pacing wires
Patients with neurostimulating devices
Patients who are TRUE claustrophobics
Patients with metallic fragments near vital structures
Patients with implanted infusion pumps
Patients with cochlear implants
Patients with motion disorders
Patients with magnetically held implants (dental, ocular)

[1] Unless ABSOLUTELY confirmed that the cerebral aneurysm clip is nonmagnetic.

the body. It is often difficult to ascertain the composition of a foreign body. An evaluation of the magnetic properties of different types of bullets has been compiled by Teitelbaum.[9] The greatest danger presented by a foreign body is a slight movement or rotation that might damage a vital structure. Before imaging a patient with a known foreign body, X-rays of the area should be obtained if there is a chance that it might lie near a major blood vessel, nerve, eye, spinal cord, or other vital structure. While most foreign bodies will move only slightly when placed in the magnetic field, a major concern with metallic foreign bodies near the eye is that there is very little resistance to movement, and a real possibility of severe injury to the retina or optic nerve. If a patient is thought to have a metallic fragment near the eye, an orbital X-ray should be obtained. If a metallic density is observed near the orbit, an MRI exam is contraindicated.

Surface coils and ECG leads are constantly used in MR images. Since they are metallic, they have the potential to cause problems, even if they are made of nonmagnetic metals. Two potential medical problems can be associated with the changing magnetic fields and deposition of rf energy occurring during a scan. First, rf energy will heat metal much more rapidly than biological tissue, so the potential exists for external metallic objects to become quite hot. These can cause heating burns. It must be emphasized that no bare metal from an ECG lead or surface coil should *ever* be allowed to contact a patient's skin. Internal metallic objects are not subject to as intense a concentration of rf energy, and heating is not a problem, although a subcutaneous metallic foreign body can cause patient discomfort, either from heating or slight motion. In a similar category are tattoos and permanent eyeliner, both of which use metallic-based dyes. The potential for heating in these areas exists, and such patients should be made aware of it.

The second potential problem associated with surface coils and ECG leads is rf or electrical burns. If a loop of electrical conductor (usually a wire) is placed in a changing magnetic field, an electrical current is induced within it. If a patient's skin is in contact with metal at two points, the patient can become part of this loop and receive a severe electrical burn. Burns can occur if the skin is directly touching any two of the following: an ECG lead; metal from a surface coil; or wire from a noninsulated portion of a surface coil cable or ECG cable. In order to prevent this from occurring, no metal from a surface coil, ECG lead, or any cable should ever be allowed to directly touch the skin of a patient. A surface coil or the head coil should never be left in the magnet when another surface coil (or the body coil) is in use. Wires should not be allowed to loop or to cross, especially underneath the patient. Cable insulation should be checked regularly for breaks in the insulation. Only cables that are electrically and thermally insulated should be used. Always be sure that an insulating pad, sponge, sheet, or the like is between the patient and any surface coil or cable. Never permit a cable to cross a surface coil.

SEDATED PATIENTS

When the need for sedation arises, vital signs of patients must be monitored. MRI-compatible systems are available to monitor patient heart rate, ECG, respiratory rate, temperature, blood pressure, and oxygen saturation. Only completely compatible systems can be used because of the potential for patient harm and equipment malfunction in the magnetic environment. MR-compatible ventilators, which are not affected by the magnetic field and do not produce image artifacts, are now available for patients requiring respiratory assistance.

QUENCHING

A quench can be defined as a loss of superconductivity. It can occur under controlled conditions, to shut the magnet down so that changes can be made, or it can occur suddenly and unexpectedly, which can be extremely hazardous. When superconductivity is lost, the magnet behaves as a resistive magnet and generates heat. The heat boils off the liquid helium and produces large amounts of helium gas. All MR-scanning rooms for superconducting magnets have to be well vented, both to vent the small amount of helium normally given off and to vent the extremely large amount of helium gas that is generated in a quench. If the helium gas is produced faster than it can be vented, it will reduce the amount of oxygen in the room by displacing it, thus making it difficult, if not impossible, to breathe. This oxygen displacement obviously could lead to a very dangerous situation if someone were caught in the scanning room, and so a rapid, unexpected quench is considered an emergency situation: All patients and personnel are required to vacate the area immediately. Quench alarms and oxygen monitors are usually placed in all superconducting magnet rooms to alert everyone around.

MRI systems are designed to be inherently safe, but detailed education of the staff is essential if the unit is to remain a safe area. Not only the technical and medical staff, but secretarial, administrative, and custodial staffs as well have to know what can and cannot be done in the vicinity of the magnet. Custodial personnel especially must be made aware of the inherent dangers involved in bringing inappropriate equipment into the room. If possible, all cleaning, deliveries, and repairs in the vicinity of the magnet room should be done under the supervision of experienced personnel. Patients should also be educated before they enter the magnet room. They should be told what to expect and what can and cannot be brought into the scanning room, and they should be questioned again about possible conditions that may prevent them from having the study (Table 9–3). Signs should be posted on the doors to scanning rooms to serve as a final reminder to patients and staff of the potential hazards of the magnetic surroundings. The importance of safety education cannot be underestimated. Only an alert staff with a thorough knowledge of proper procedures will ensure safe and effective examinations.

POINTS TO PONDER

- Stationary magnetic fields of up to 2.0 T are considered safe to humans.

- The specific absorption rate (SAR) is the rate at which energy is absorbed by tissue.

- MR imaging is considered safe by the FDA for all patients except those with pacemakers, neurostimulating devices, and cerebral aneurysm clips.

- MR imaging of pregnant patients has been neither approved nor disapproved by the FDA and is still under investigation.

- MR imaging may be used in pregnant women if other non-ionizing forms of diagnostic imaging are inadequate or if the examination provides important information that would otherwise require exposure to ionizing radiation (e.g., fluoroscopy, CT).

- No deleterious effects of static MR fields have been demonstrated for pregnant MR technologists, physicians, and nurses.

- Pregnant MR workers should not remain in the room while the actual scanning is being performed.

- Gradients are responsible for the loud knocking or banging noises associated with MR scanning.

- Earplugs should be given to all patients.

- Noise produced during the examination is considerably below a level of concern for any permanent auditory effects.

- Hearing aids must be removed before scanning.

- Gadolinium is a paramagnetic substance that, when combined with various chelating agents, is safe for use in normal patients.

- Concern about the use of gadolinium exists for pregnant patients and patients with impaired renal function.

- The missile effect, in which loose metallic objects are pulled forcibly toward the magnet, can be dangerous, even with small objects.

POINTS TO PONDER *(continued)*

- Patients with implanted electronic, magnetic, or mechanical metallic devices are not candidates for MR examinations.

- Absolute verification must be made that a patient's implanted aneurysm clip is nonmagnetic before he or she is scanned.

- The location of a metallic foreign body should be determined with X-rays to be sure that it is not near a vital structure.

- Temperature burns can occur if the patient's skin is in direct contact with a piece of metal.

- Electrical burns can occur if the patient is in contact with metal at two points and becomes part of an electrical loop in the changing magnetic field.

- Vital signs of sedated patients should always be monitored.

- A quench results in a loss of superconductivity, increase in temperature, and rapid boil-off of liquid helium.

- Education of the staff and patients as to proper safety procedures is essential for the safe and effective operation of an MR facility.

REFERENCES

1. Shellock FG, Kanal E. *Magnetic Resonance: Bioeffects, Safety, and Patient Management.* New York: Raven Press; 1994: 46–47.
2. Kanal E, Shellock FG, Sonnenblick D. MRI clinical site safety survey: Phase I results and preliminary data. *Magn Reson Imag.* 1988; 7: 106.
3. Shellock FG, Kanal E. Policies, guidelines, and recommendations for MR imaging safety and patient management. *J Magn Reson Imag.* 1991; 1: 97.
4. Kanal E, Gillen J, Evans J, Savitz D, Shellock FG. Survey of reproductive health among female MR workers. *Radiology.* 1993; 187: 395–399.
5. Shellock and Kanal, 1994: 46.
6. Brummett RE, Talbot JM, Charuhas P. Potential hearing loss resulting from MR imaging. *Radiology.* 1988; 169: 539–540.

7. Goldman AM, Gossman WE, Friedlander PC. Reduction of sound levels with antinoise in MR imaging. *Radiology.* 1989; 173: 549–550.
8. Klucznik RP, Carrier DA, Pyka R, Haid RW. Placement of a ferromagnetic intracerebral aneurysm clip in a magnetic field with a fatal outcome. *Radiology.* 1993; 187: 855–856.
9. Teitelbaum GP, Yee CA, Van Horn DD, Kim HS, Colletti PM. Metallic ballistic fragments: MR imaging safety and artifacts. *Radiology.* June 1990; 175(3): 855–859.

CHAPTER TEN

IDENTIFYING AND MINIMIZING IMAGE ARTIFACTS

Image artifacts are associated with every radiologic imaging modality. Motion blurring on plain films, metallic star artifacts or detector-imbalance ring artifacts on CT scans, and refraction image distortion on ultrasound studies are but a few well documented examples in radiology. In terms of the MR image, an artifact is an abnormal area of signal within the image that does not arise from patient anatomy or pathology. It is a "false" signal: While the signal is real, it does not arise from the actual patient tissues. It is important to recognize artifacts for two important reasons: first, to eliminate diagnostic error, when the artifact hides or falsely suggests a pathologic condition, and second, to recognize that certain artifacts can indicate particular problems within the system itself so that proper service or repair can be started before major problems occur.

In general, all artifacts fall into four categories: (1) those associated with the patient; (2) those associated with physiology; (3) those inherent in the principles of MR imaging; and (4) those associated with the hardware and software of the imaging system. As newer pulse sequences continue to be developed, new artifacts can be produced and known artifacts can result from multiple causes, making the precise classification of these eccentricities more difficult.

Artifacts associated with the patient are normally due to random movement or metallic objects (either external or internal) that distort the image, and physiological artifacts are produced by breathing, cardiac or peristaltic motion, and blood flow. The imaging system produces artifacts that result either from the basic physical principles of MRI (chemical shift and flow) or from instrumental factors (rf, gradients, shims, or computer hardware). Although the most obvious artifacts can often be attributed to the patient, some suggestion of instrumental artifacts is present in almost all imaging situations (depending upon the pulse sequences and stability of the hardware). Most such artifacts manifest themselves in the direction of the phase-encoding gradients by combinations of rings, streaks, and ghosting that could either be patient or instrument based. Table 10–1 at the end of this chapter lists the various types of artifacts observed, the methods of determining the type of artifact encountered, and ways of eliminating artifacts. The development of a practical quality-assurance program for monitoring system performance and for efficiently using the manufacturer's field service and engineering staff is strongly dependent on the recognition and characterization of the image artifacts listed in this table.

TYPES OF ARTIFACTS

A. Artifacts Resulting from the Patient

Patient-related artifacts are almost always caused either by something the patient is doing (usually moving) or by something out of the ordinary that the patient has inside or outside of the body. The most common patient-caused artifact is motion during data acquisition. Motion artifacts are always propagated in the phase-encoding direction. Random patient motion appears as a blurring of the image (Figure 10–1).

Random patient movements can be minimized by either sedation or patient education and cooperation. Patients who are unable to cooperate by lying still during the examination require sedation. These patients include those suffering from dementia, motion disorders, or extreme claustrophobia. Explaining the procedure to the patient and emphasizing the necessity to lie still is usually sufficient to ensure cooperation. Children or nervous patients may require additional reassurance by having someone in the room with them during the examination. If motion persists, taping or using Velcro straps to hold the body part secure partially immobilizes the area of interest and serves as a reminder to the patient to remain still.

Nonbiologic materials in or on the patient cause different types of artifacts, depending upon the composition of the specific object. These items can be classified as either metallic or nonmetallic. Some nonmetallic materials have mobile hydrogen atoms associated with them, others do not. If they do not have mobile hydrogen atoms, the objects will simply produce a signal void (no signal). Should there be a large difference in magnetic susceptibilities, such as with air and water, a susceptibility artifact will be produced. This will appear as a rim of high signal around the edge of the region of signal void (Figure 10–2). If the material does have mobile protons, it will produce the appropriate signal for the type of material that it is.

Metallic objects can be categorized as nonmagnetic, slightly magnetic (or magnetizable), or highly magnetic. Nonmagnetic objects carried or worn outside of the body will not affect the scan. Nonmagnetic objects inside the body (prostheses, surgical clips, sutures, valves, plates, etc.) will simply produce a region devoid of signal corresponding to the object, but they will not distort the image outside this region.

Objects that are slightly magnetic or magnetizable will cause a small region of magnetic distortion around the device. Note that patients can be scanned even if known magnetic implants are present, since valuable diagnostic information can

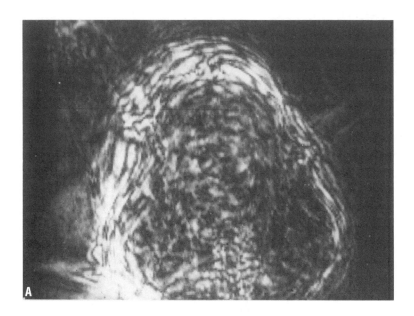

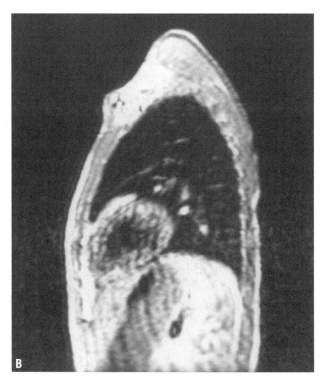

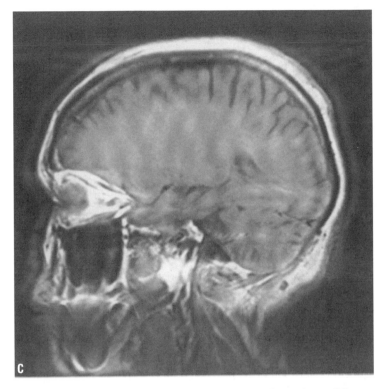

Figure 10–1. Various degrees of motion will produce different grades of artifact: (A) Inability of patient to cooperate at all leads to a completely uninterpretable axial image of the head. (B) Slight motion during the scan significantly decreases the resolution of this sagittal image of the chest. (C) This patient having a head scan was sneezing during the sagittal acquisition.

often be obtained in regions not obscured by the foreign body. Such implants often produce a region of greatly enhanced signal around the periphery of the object. Since the most intense pixel in an image is part of the algorithm for allocating the gray scale, the effect of having a metallic object that produces an increase in regional signal intensity (often by a factor of 10 or more) is to severely limit the available gray scale for the rest of the image, producing a so-called washed-out image. Most implanted devices will experience minimal interactions with the magnetic field. We have not found any rf, gradient, or any other potential side-

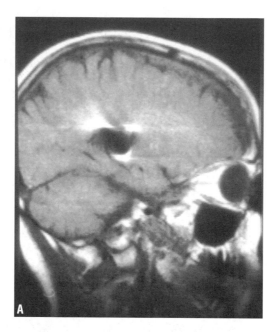

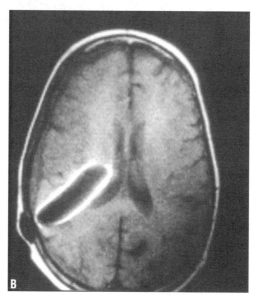

Figure 10–2. (A) Sagittal and (B) axial images through the head of a patient with a ventricular shunt. Note the high-intensity signal artifact at the edges of the shunt due to susceptibility effects.

effect to be at all significant with any prosthetic device. Because of possible effects of the magnetic fields on physiologic pacing devices or cerebral aneurysm clips, however, patients who have these devices are not scanned.

In those situations where the metallic object is highly magnetic, there will be significant distortion of the images, sometimes sufficient to render the study completely nondiagnostic (Figure 10–3). More often, however, much useful information can be obtained even though part of the anatomy cannot be evaluated because of the metallic artifact.

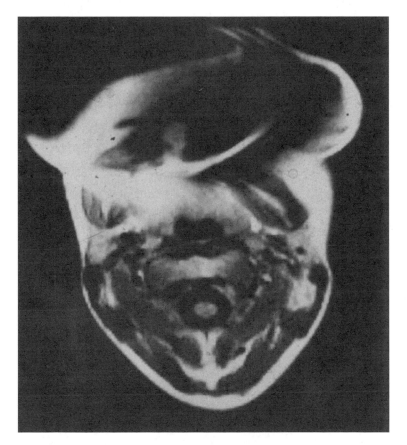

Figure 10–3. The anterior portion of inferior head is obscured by severe magnetic distortion from a nonremovable dental bridge. Note that the posterior portion, including the spinal cord, is well visualized.

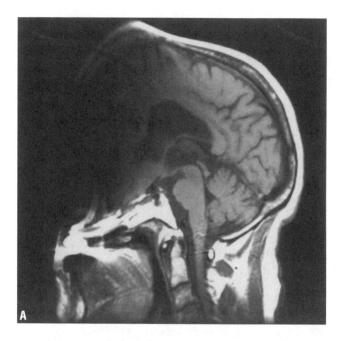

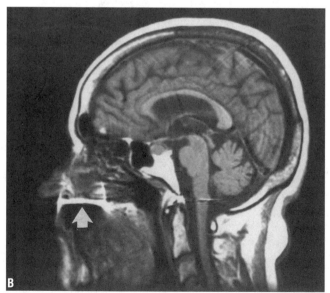

Figure 10–4.   (A) Marked distortion of the sagittal image of the head due to the patient's failure to remove a hair pin. (B) Image after the hair pin was removed. Note that the metallic artifact due to a dental prosthesis (arrow) is still present.

Personal articles such as dentures, keys, jewelry, hair pins, snaps, and belt buckles will produce artifacts that may either cause local signal enhancement at the periphery of the object or effectively (if magnetic) distort part or all of the image (Figure 10–4). Careful attention by the interviewing staff, patient education through appropriate interviews and questionnaires, and alert technologists can minimize these artifacts.

Of considerable interest and of increasing importance is the fact that new types of highly colored make-up (especially certain types of mascara containing ferromagnetic compounds) will cause magnetic artifacts (Figure 10–5). Tattoos, as mentioned in Chapter 9, contain dyes that have magnetic materials in them. The artifacts that they produce will be relatively small and on the surface of the skin. Technologists observing that a patient has a tattoo

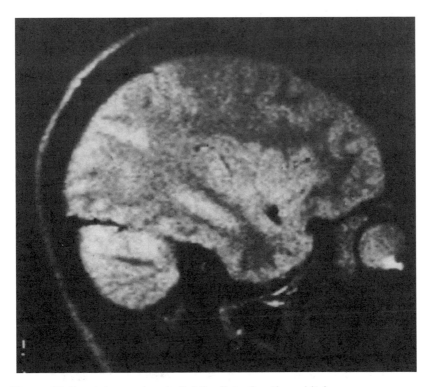

Figure 10–5.   Intense signal slightly distorting the orbit from mascara containing ferromagnetic compounds.

should make a note of it so that the radiologist will be aware of the source of the abnormality. More serious than the artifact problem is the fact that, especially with the new fast-scanning techniques, tattooed regions may heat up because of excessive rf deposition in the metals and cause discomfort to the patient. Patients should be made aware of this fact, and sufficient time should be allowed for energy radiation between scans. In other words, these patients should be scanned more slowly than normal to ensure that no heating occurs. Artifacts must always be considered as a possible explanation when image abnormalities are observed.

B. Physiology-Related Artifacts

Physiologic motions are generally a more common source of arti- facts that are voluntary movements. Physiologic motions are observed more in the body than in the head, since the only physi- ologic motions to produce artifacts in the head are blood flow and CSF pulsation. Artifacts due to a continuous or periodic motion, as occurs with respiration, cardiac pulsation, or blood flow, can be recognized as image blurring with ringed structures around and through the image in the direction of the phase-encoding gradient direction (Figure 10–6). These ringed signals appear in "space," the

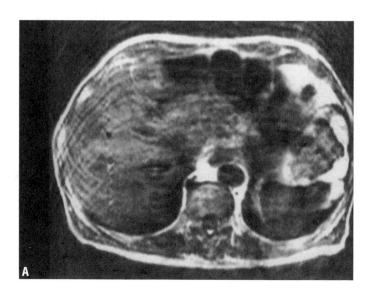

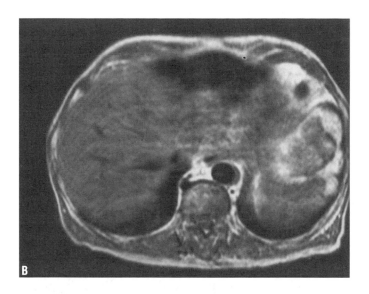

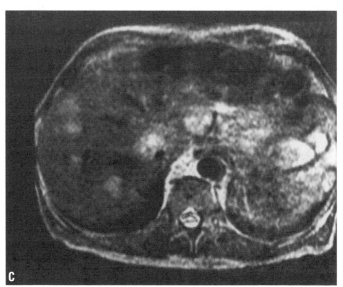

Figure 10–6.   (A) Proton-density axial image through the abdomen, demonstrating a ghosting artifact ringing through and above the image, which produces significant loss of motion and uninterpretable T2-weighted image. (B) Same section as in A except that respiratory compensation was applied, allowing multiple lesions to be observed in the liver on the T2-weighted image (C).

empty area in the bore of the magnet where there is no tissue, as if they were ghosts; this type of artifact is referred to as **ghosting**.

Respiratory motion blurs image details and produces displaced signal artifacts in images of the chest, the abdomen, and sometimes the pelvis as well. These artifacts will be projected in the direction of the phase-encoding direction, and usually, as long as they are recognized, will not interfere with image interpretation. On occasion there will be a problem, which can usually be solved by repeating the sequence after switching the phase-encoding direction (Figure 8–12). In Chapter 8 we discussed the effects of respiratory and cardiac motion and methods of reducing them. More subtle motion effects are produced by the peristaltic activity of the bowel. Peristalsis is rarely sufficient to produce ghosting, so only a subtle blurring in the region of the bowel is observed, without effect on other structures. Administration of glucagon has been utilized to stop peristalsis with questionable success; however, fast scanning techniques are now capable of greatly reducing bowel-motion effects.

Cardiac motion blurs image details in the neighborhood of the heart and produces a characteristic column of displaced signal equal to the width of the heart, observed in the phase-encoding direction. ECG-gating techniques usually improve images of the heart quite satisfactorily, and new fast scanning techniques capture cardiac images so rapidly that they are not degraded by motion (Figure 10–7).

The production of artifacts in an image due to flow is a complex subject, since many different factors can contribute to the appearance of flowing blood. It is impossible to eliminate most of these artifacts, so recognition of them is essential in order to make a proper diagnosis. The most usual appearance of flowing blood—no signal at all—can technically be considered an artifact, since there is blood there, but it is not producing a signal (Figure 10–8). As previously discussed, although the volume of blood within the section being imaged receives the initial 90° pulse, it has left the imaging plane before it can experience the refocusing pulse. Thus, under "normal" conditions flowing blood produces no signal, referred to as a "flow void." If, however, the blood is moving slowly enough, some of it may still be within the imaging region when the refocusing pulse is applied, and this blood may produce a

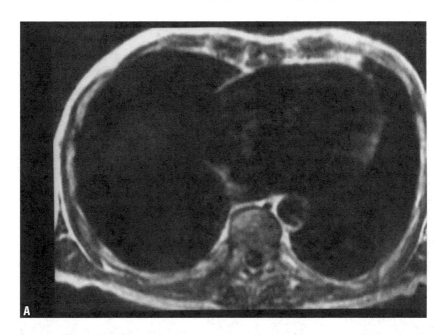

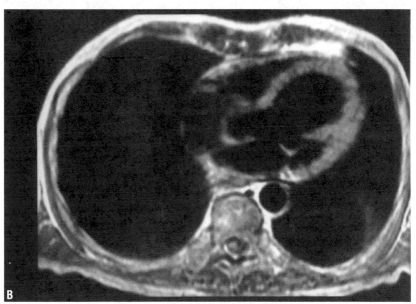

Figure 10–7.   (A) Nongated image of the chest shows blurring of the cardiac chambers. (B) ECG-gated image through the same section improves resolution notably.

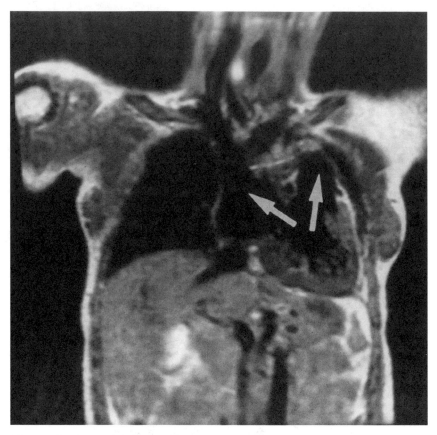

Figure 10–8. Normal blood flow (arrows) leaves a signal void as it flows through the aorta and pulmonary artery from a common ventricle, in this congenital heart variation.

signal. This type of artifact is appropriately called a "slow flow" artifact, or paradoxical enhancement. In tortuous vessels, or areas near a constriction, blood flow may not be uniform, but it can be turbulent (Figure 10–9). In turbulent flow the blood swirls around and back, eventually moving forward. Areas of turbulence will produce patchy and irregular signal within the lumen of the blood vessel. If the scan is repeated, the pattern will change, indicating that it is an artifact and not thrombus or plaque within the vessel; if a multi-echo sequence is used, the pattern will not remain constant, since the refocusing pulse for the second echo occurs after the blood has continued moving or swirling.

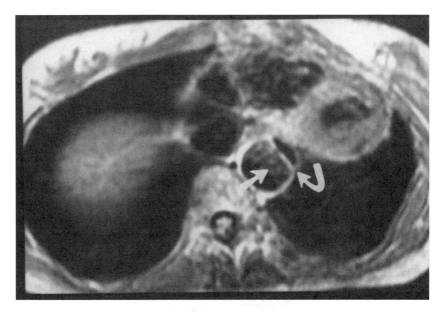

Figure 10–9. Turbulent flow (arrow) is observed in the lumen of this descending aorta. The intimal flap (curved arrow), which separates the true lumen from the false lumen in this descending, is well seen.

When blood remains in the imaging plane long enough to receive the refocusing pulse, another type of enhancement can occur for sections imaged during diastole in an ECG-gated study. Since blood flow is pulsatile, more so in arteries than in veins, during diastole blood will be relatively stationary and will emit a signal (Figure 10–10). The signal will be stronger at shorter repetition times. If the vessel is not perpendicular to the imaging plane (oblique sectioning of vessels), increased signal on the downstream edge of the oblique section is obtained, which can easily be confused with plaque or thrombus. In such cases an MRA or confirmation by observation in another imaging plane should be obtained. During a multi-echo acquisition in a spin-echo sequence, if echoes are obtained as multiples of the echo time (30 ms, 60 ms, 90 ms, etc.) nuclei that are out of phase (no signal) during acquisition of the first echo (30 ms) will be in phase (positive signal) 30 ms later, at 60 ms, when the second echo is acquired. This is easily recognized, since blood exhibits a normal flow void on odd-numbered echoes and produces a signal on even-numbered echoes.

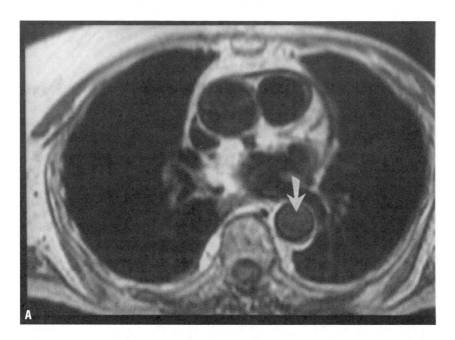

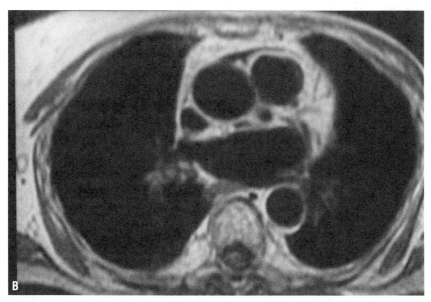

Figure 10–10.   (A) Signal is observed in the descending aorta (arrow) in this section obtained during late diastole, while in the adjacent slice (B), obtained during early diastole, the aorta is free of signal.

C. Artifacts Caused by Instrumental Effects

A problem with any one of the many components of an MRI system can cause a problem with the final image; it is therefore easy to see that a great many types of image artifacts are caused by instrumentation. These artifacts can be created during data acquisition, data processing, image display, or filming. The two most easily corrected artifacts are those arising from display and filming, since these processes can be repeated very easily by redisplaying or refilming.

Most instrumental artifacts arise during data acquisition. The high-powered analog circuits necessary for data acquisition are much less reliable than the low-powered digital circuits used for data processing. These artifacts usually cannot be eliminated, and a new data set must be obtained after repairs have been effected. Changes in magnetic fields can present problems: resistive magnets can have power-supply problems; permanent magnets can have thermal problems; superconductive magnets can decay slowly or quench rapidly.

Most commonly, however, magnetic field artifacts result from problems with shims. The shims control multiple independent coils, and only one of these channels will fail at any given time. Depending upon which channel fails, the resulting spatial distortion in the image may be obvious or quite subtle; it may be more obvious in one imaging plane than another. These types of artifacts will usually be more evident in the body coil because of the larger field of view. They will appear as either a geometric distortion, usually due to a failure of the shim power supply, or fine ghosting due to shim-gradient interactions (Figure 10–11). The problem can usually be corrected by checking the shim power supply, the shim settings, or the isolation circuits.

Gradient instabilities will produce blurring and loss of resolution, which may be subtle at times (Figure 10–12). These instabilities can result from thermal overloads (which occur easily if the air conditioning isn't functioning properly). The shim-gradient interactions that are produced by failures in the shim isolation circuits can progress to "singing" oscillations (oscillations in the audible range), which can be heard. Image banding can occur with a coupling of eddy currents to the

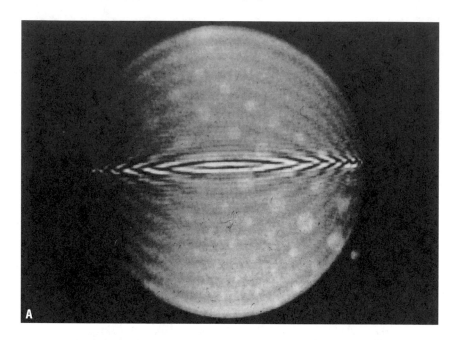

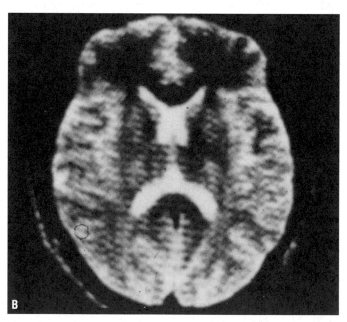

Figure 10–11. (A) Geometric misrepresentation of a uniformly filled circular phantom due to gradient overheating. (B) Gradient overheating causing motion-like artifact; however, the clarity of cerebral structures in this case should be contrasted with the general blurring observed when patient motion is present.

gradient and rf body coil, especially in multi-echo sequences. This artifact is difficult to correct completely, but it may be remedied by checking and retuning the eddy current circuits. Truncation and aliasing can be corrected by using more phase-encoding steps.

Radiofrequency problems can also occur. Discrete lines or streaks through the image are signs of an rf-shielding leak, or possibly an rf source coming from within the magnet room, Fluorescent light bulbs that are just about to burn out are a notorious cause of rf interference; as a result, most scanning rooms no longer utilize fluorescent lighting (Figure 10–13). Instabilities in the rf transmitter produce ghosting patterns, or a "zipper" artifact. Decreased signal or increased noise can result from rf amplifier failure, improper tip angles, or incorrect matching of the impedance of coils to preamps. Highly nonuniform images are produced by rf coil inhomogeneities and by inclusion or reconstruction artifacts. Unless properly tuned, surface coils can receive so much signal from subcutaneous fat that the rest of the image may be compressed into the gray scale near the noise level. This can be corrected by adjusting the field of view to eliminate the subcutaneous tissue or by renormalizing the image.

After the analog signal has been converted to a digital format, the digitized image data is processed. This opens up a whole new category of artifacts: those produced during data processing (Figure 10–14). All of these artifacts can be eliminated by reprocessing the image data, *if* it has not yet been deleted from the disk. Errors can be caused by a bit-drop, which can produce a herringbone effect, or if more severe, reduce the entire image to a geometric banding, or cause moiré patterns or variable patterns (Figure 10–15). As data is transferred from one part of the computer to another, data transfer artifacts will be produced. Array processor errors may affect only one image in a series, or may corrupt an entire series, distorting them or turning them into geometric patterns (Figure 10–16).

D. Artifacts Inherent in the Imaging Process
Several different types of artifacts can occur because of the very nature of the magnetic resonance imaging procedure. The most important of these is called **aliasing**, or wrap-around.

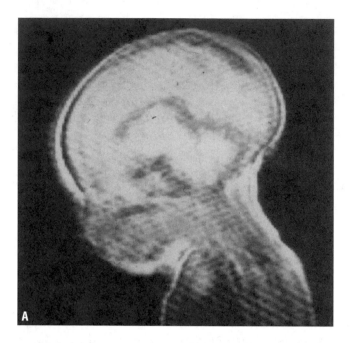

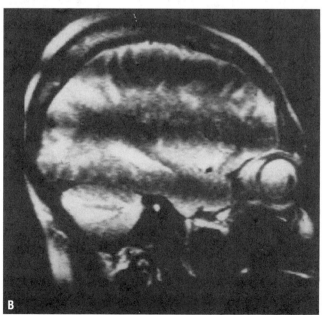

Figure 10–12. (A) Fine ghosting produced by gradient overheating. (B) Image banding caused in part by eddy current-gradient interaction. (C) Herringbone pattern throughout the image and background. (D) Complete gradient failure.

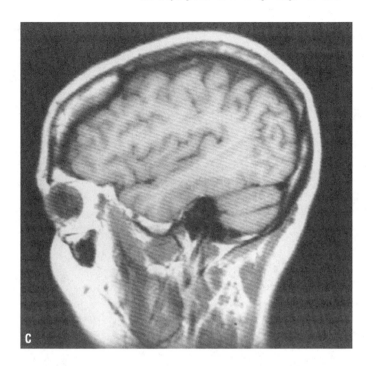

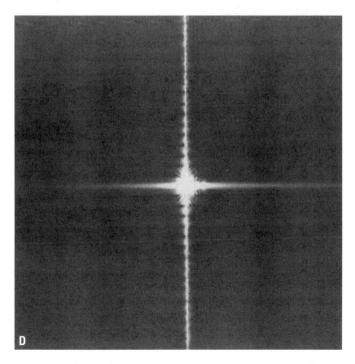

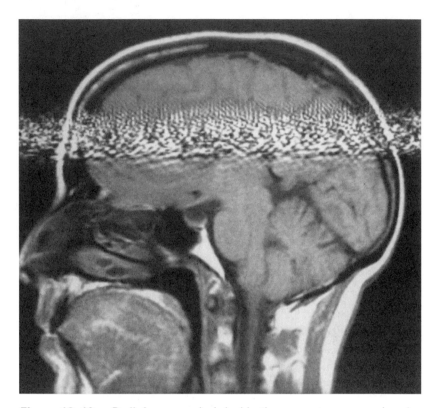

Figure 10–13. Radiofrequency leak inside the magnet room produced a band of rf artifact through the affected frequency range in the frequency-encoding direction.

This refers to a situation in which the edge of the left side of the object is superimposed on the right side of the image, and vice versa. If the part of the body being imaged extends outside of the field of view, a signal from these "excluded" tissues still will be produced. This can occur in both the frequency-encoding direction and the phase-encoding direction. Digital rf filters can eliminate the wrap-around effect in the frequency-encoding direction by providing a sharp cutoff of signal frequency at the edges of the field of view in the directions of the frequency-encoding gradient. In the phase-encoding direction, however, no such filter exists. If part of the anatomy extends outside of the field of view in the phase-encoding

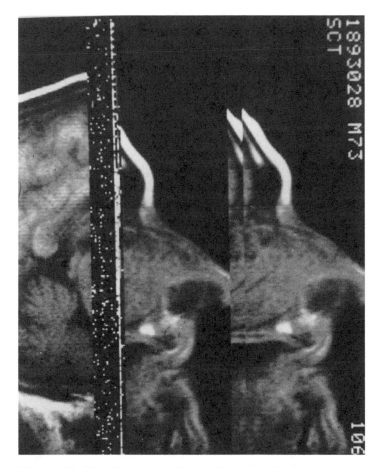

Figure 10–14. Reconstruction artifacts producing improper superimposition of several parts of an image.

direction, it experiences a phase shift that is similar to a point on the opposite side of the anatomy. It will emit a signal, then, that is identical to signal from the other side (see Figure 10–17). In order to avoid this, the number of phase-encoding steps is increased, but only the area of interest is reconstructed. This is called **oversampling**. The FOV is increased and the pixel size is kept the same so as not to diminish resolution in the image. This requires the number of phase-encoding steps to be increased. Only the central pixels are reconstructed, and

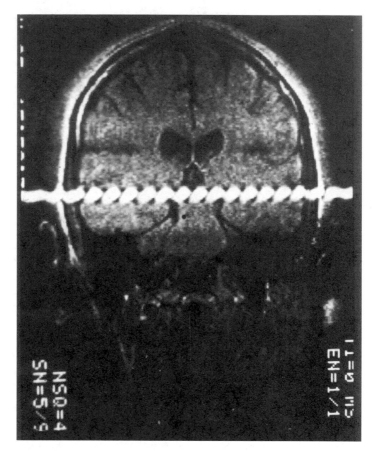

Figure 10–15.   A bit-drop artifact produced an unusual addition to a coronal view of the head.

although aliasing will still occur, it will produce an artifact in a region that is not going to be reconstructed, and thus will not appear in the image (Figure 10–17D). This is an option called "no phase wrap." It increases the area being imaged and also increases the imaging time or reduces the number of slices available for imaging. Since it does limit several options, it should be used only if anatomy extends beyond the field of view in the phase-encoding direction.

During an MRI examination, we are imaging mobile protons in the body. Essentially, there are two different types:

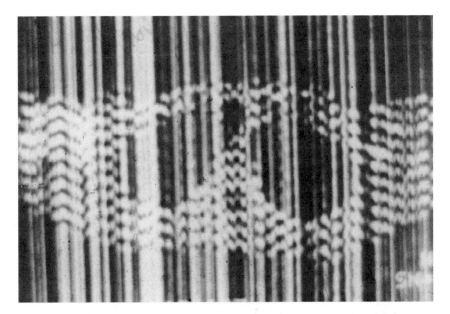

Figure 10–16. Array processor malfunction in an axial image of the chest.

protons associated with water (essentially in soft tissue) and protons associated with fat. Although their signals are very close to each other, they are not identical. There is a difference in frequency (frequency shift) due to the differences in chemical nature of the two types of protons. The fat signal appears at 3.7 ppm downfield (at the lower end) from the soft tissue signal. At 1.5 T this amounts to a difference of about 240 Hz. This variance is small when considering that we are imaging at approximately 63 MHz, but it can have noticeable effects. The difference at 0.3 T would be 48 Hz, so the chemical shift effects are much more pronounced at higher field strengths. The effect is noticeable only at a boundary between soft tissue and fat (Figure 10–18). The fat that we observe in an image is actually produced 3.7 ppm upfield (the signal is shifted 3.7 ppm downfield).

When fat is surrounded by soft tissues, a dark band appears at the upfield interface and a bright band appears at the downfield interface of the fatty region. The dark band results from the fat signal being shifted downfield and leaving behind a signal

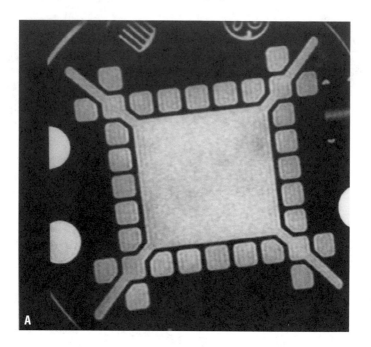

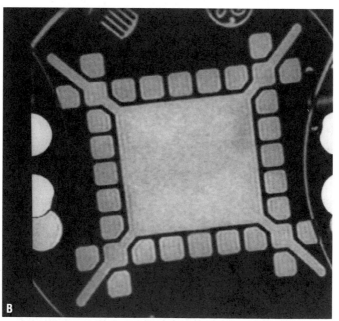

Figure 10–17. (A) This is an example of a proper image of a phantom at a small FOV using an oversampling technique. (B) If the oversampling correction is not employed, aliasing is observed in the phase-encoding direction.

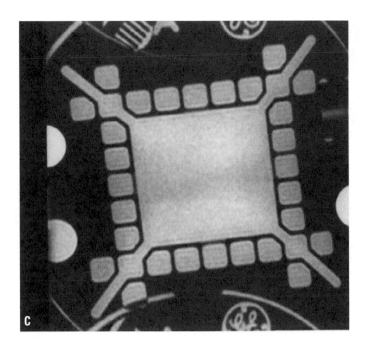

phase-encoding direction

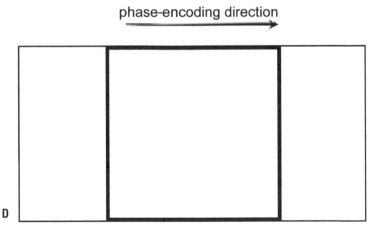

Figure 10–17. *(cont.)*   (C) By reversing the phase and frequency directions, the aliasing artifact is switched, always remaining in the direction of the phase-encoding gradient. (D) A 256-by-256 matrix has been prescribed, with the no phase wrap, or oversampling option. The area of interest is contained in the central square (heavy lined box) but the area being scanned is outlined by the thinner lines. This additional area extends outward in the phase-encoding direction. Any aliasing artifact will appear in these outer boxes, but since only the central area is reconstructed there will not be an aliasing artifact in the image.

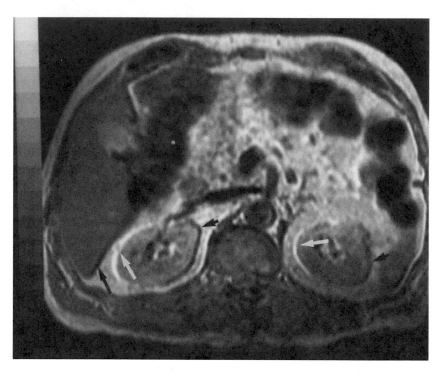

Figure 10–18.   Chemical shift artifact demonstrated as a rim of decreased signal at the fat/soft-tissue interfaces on the right sides of both kidneys and the liver (black arrows), and as a rim of increased signal on the left sides of both kidneys (white arrows).

void. The bright band results from the fat signal being shifted downfield and adding to the soft tissue signal already present.

When soft tissues are surrounded by fat, a bright band appears at the upfield interface and a dark band appears at the downfield interface of the soft tissue region. The bright band results from the fat signal being shifted downfield and reenforcing the soft tissue signal already present. The dark band downfield results from the fat signal being shifted downfield and leaving behind a signal void.

Magnetic susceptibility is the ability of a material to become magnetized when placed in a magnetic field. This may cause a distortion in the local magnetic field and may also cause artifacts. Local variations in susceptibility, T2* effects, will cause regions of signal void with an intensely bright signal at the region of the interface. T2* effects are usually caused by a metallic foreign body, but iron from a hemorrhage can cause a similar effect. Gradient-echo images are very sensitive to changes in susceptibility, and T2* effects can be magnified on these images (Figure 10–19).

Chemical shift and T2* susceptibility artifacts are proof that the difference between an artifact and a diagnostic sign can fool

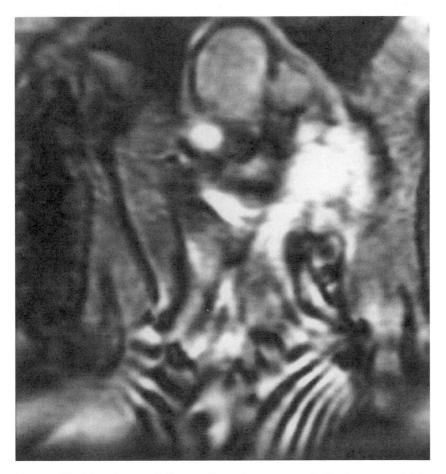

Figure 10–19. Susceptibility artifact due to surgical clips completely obscures this gradient-echo image of the abdomen.

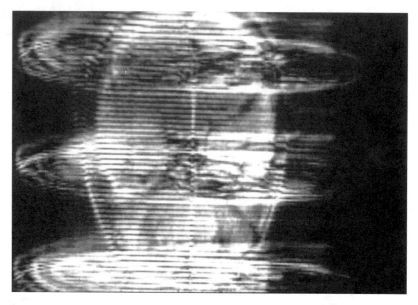

Figure 10–20. Strange yet artistic artifact from as-yet-undetermined multiple causes.

even the most experienced eye, if the existence artifacts are not kept in mind. There have been efforts both to suppress and to exploit both of these effects.

Some of the many different causes of image artifacts can be avoided by proper screening of patients, making sure that they do not have removable metal objects with them. Note should be made of any surgical appliances within the body, so they can be taken into account when interpreting the scan. Instrumental artifacts can be recognized and corrected, or with proper quality assurance can be anticipated and avoided. Recognizing and understanding artifacts is important to the production and interpretation of images, and eventually to patient welfare (Figure 10–20).

POINTS TO PONDER

- Artifacts are signals in the image that do not represent signal from the patient's biological tissues.

- Artifacts can be caused by the patient or objects with the patient, by physiologic motion, or by the components of the imaging system, or they can be intrinsic to the basic concepts of MRI.

- Proper screening of patients will eliminate a large portion of potential artifacts.

- Familiarity with and recognition of artifacts is of primary importance to a proper interpretation of an MRI examination.

TABLE 10–1. CLASSIFICATION, SOURCES, AND CORRECTION OF ARTIFACTS

Source	Artifact	Remedy	Comments
A. Patient-Related Artifacts			
Uncontrolled/random movement	Image blurring with displaced signal	Patient education/cooperation. Small children and some adults may need sedation.	Certain conditions preclude patients from having MRIs (tremors, dementia, severe claustrophobia).
Foreign materials in or on body			
No mobile protons (nonmetallic)	Lack of signal in the area—no signal distortion	No correction necessary—recognition important.	Patient images not affected.
Sudden changes in magnetic susceptibility	Significantly increased rim of intensity around substance	Remove object if possible.	Recognition important.
Metallic objects (surgical implants)	Image will be distorted around the object, with the degree of distortion dependent upon the magnetic properties of the metal	Recognize as artifact.	Valuable diagnostic information can be obtained even from distorted images; re-normalization of gray scale may be necessary for intensely bright metallic artifacts; patients with pacemakers and cerebral aneurysm clips not scanned.
Metallic objects (personal)	Metallic distortion, as above	Removal eliminates artifact.	Coins, keys, jewelry, clips, buckles, etc., not a problem if patient asked to remove them, or if patient is gowned. Hairpins always potential problem because of reluctance to remove them. Dentures should be removed for head and neck scans, if possible.

Cosmetics	Ferromagnetic-based (usually highly colored), will produce local distortions	Mascara most common offender.
Tattoos and permanently applied eyeliner	Local distortion	Heating effects may occur which will be uncomfortable and patients should be warned in advance.
B. Physiologic Artifacts		
Respiration	Image blurring; ghosting, displaced signal around and through image along the phase-encoding direction	Respiratory gating or compensation usually effective in reducing (not eliminating) effect; fast scan techniques with breath holding very useful; anterior saturation pulses also helpful. Compensation will reduce ghosting but less effective with image blurring.
Cardiac motion	Ghosting observed over width of heart in and out of the chest in the direction of the phase-encoding gradient; loss of resolution of cardiac and other mediastinal structures	ECG gating reduces ghosting and image blurring, scanning time reduced. T1 contrast modulated by heart rate.
Peristalsis	Blurring of bowel and surrounding structures; most conspicuous in anterior abdomen	Glucagon has been suggested but is of questionable practical value; fast scanning techniques are promising.
Flow	Absent signal	Elimination of these artifacts is usually not possible so recognition is key to the proper interpretive response.
Rapid flow		

(continued)

215

TABLE 10–1. *(continued)*

Source	Artifact	Remedy	Comments
	Decreased flow rate	Increased signal possible	
	Even echo enhancement	Increased signal on even-numbered echoes	
	Diastolic pseudogating	Increased signal on slices obtained during diastole	Caused by ECG gating.
	Turbulence	Both increased and decreased signals observed	Pattern not consistent if scan repeated.	Pattern not consistent if multiple echoes obtained.
	Oblique sectioning of vessels	Increased signal on downstream side of vessel		Easily confused with plaque or thrombus; confirmation in additional plane necessary.
	Diffusion	Odd/even echo alternations		

C. Artifacts Inherent in the Imaging Process

Source	Artifact	Remedy	Comments
Chemical shift		Inclusion of fat signal in soft tissue pixels at fat/soft tissue interface on downfield side of frequency-encoded direction produces rim of increased signal; decreased signal on upfield side	Recognition key.	Artifact due to fat proton signal being 3 ppm lower than water proton signal.
T2* effects		Increased sensitivity to local variations in susceptibility	Eliminated by 180° pulse or by reversing gradient.	Effect permits hemorrhage to be observed earlier at lower magnetic field strengths.

D. System-Caused Artifacts

Source	Artifact	Remedy	Comments
Gradients		Periodic blurring in phase-encoding direction	Overheating (problem with air conditioning or water cooling circuit); replace transistors in gradient drivers.	Easily confused with patient motion; can be checked on imaging phantom.

	Symptom	Correction	Cause/Comment
	Fine ghosting	Rigid securing of rf coil will minimize motion.	Due to slight motion of rf coil due to gradient drive.
	Truncation and aliasing	Use more phase-encoding gradient steps.	Different reconstruction methods may also be helpful.
	Banding	Retune or check eddy current circuits.	Caused by a coupling of eddy currents to gradient and rf body coils in multi-echo sequences; difficult to completely correct
Shims	Geometric distortion	Check shim power supply.	Usually due to shim power supply failure or incorrect shim settings.
	Ghosting from shim-gradient interactions	Check isolation circuits.	
rf effects	Discrete lines or streaks	Check rf shielding or possible rf sources in magnet room.	Local rf transmission; rf shielding leak; local rf pickup may also occur via table/magnet coupling.
	Decreased signal, increased noise	Check amplifier gain, diodes, or tip angles (perform manual tune).	rf amplifier failure; isolation diode failure; incorrect tip angles; incorrect impedance matching of coils to preamps.
	Inhomogeneities in image	Check tip angles; retune compensating gradients.	Coil or shim problems are also possible error sources.
	Image contrast changes	Check tip angles and pulse shapes.	Incorrect tip angles, pulse shapes or compensating gradients.
Computer hardware	Moiré patterns; geometrical banding; highly variable distortions	Replace appropriate computer boards.	Bit drop in data transfer.
	Miscellaneous patterns; incomplete or repetitive reconstructive patterns	Acquisition, transfer or storage errors will mean rescanning the patient; reconstruction or display errors can be corrected by software techniques.	Failures may occur during data acquisition, transfer, storage, reconstruction or display.

ROUTINE SYSTEM PROCEDURES: PHOTOGRAPHY, ARCHIVAL, AND QUALITY CONTROL

The maintenance of proper quality assurance (QA) has major technical, diagnostic, medical, and legal implications. If performed routinely and conscientiously, it will involve only the physicist, technologist, and field service personnel. If neglected, it will affect physicians, administrators, accreditation committees, and attorneys. With so many interested parties, there are divergent interpretations and expectations from QA analysis. It is important, therefore, that QA be taken as a significant and substantive procedure that should be performed meticulously on a precise schedule.

QA procedures are presumed to demonstrate how well the unit is functioning. The testing should be devised so that if a problem is detected, the analysis will provide enough information to localize the precise component that is failing. More important, the perfect QA program should also be able to provide clues to enable the physicist or technologist to predict the failure and correct it before it occurs, by detecting the more subtle problems that preceded it. If an impending defect in a particular component can be identified early, MRI personnel can perform preventive maintenance and consequently avoid losing time and money, as well as eliminating significant frustration.

Most efficient QA designs are based on careful observations of performance over time. A continual and routine acquisition of data during normal operation is essential if one is to observe a deviation from the norm. The critical question is, what details of system performance should be observed?

QA is a particularly important aspect of MRI because of both the number of variables involved and the range of information available. In addition, the contributions to image quality are much more interrelated in MRI than in other forms of medical imaging, and the technology is not only new to most medical users but also is continuing to evolve rapidly.

Which tests to perform is determined by a theoretical knowledge of which features are important to performance. How often to perform them must usually be learned through experience for each piece of equipment. Testing will also be shaped by the options available and the goals of the users. Testing should be directed towards those factors most likely to affect image quality and those factors most likely to change. The suggestions given here are indications of where to start. Specific additional testing will vary with the individual users. It is of particular importance that all QA testing be repeated after each major upgrade and repair, so that a new baseline can be established.

The most basic tool for QA in MRI is the **uniformity phantom** (Figure 11–1). This device should almost, but not completely, fill the field of view in all directions. Rectangular phantoms are sometimes preferred over circular phantoms because they fill more of the field of view (Figure 11–2). At least two different phantoms are necessary: one for the head coil and one for the body coil. They can be filled with a variety of substances. Propylene glycol, ethylene glycol, gels, and aqueous solutions have all been used, as well as many phantoms with several components, to produce areas of different signal intensities. A

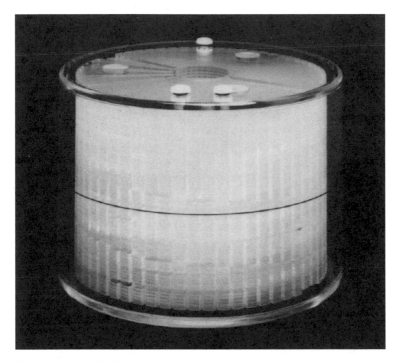

Figure 11–1.   STC Phantom for measuring slice thickness, contiguity, and position. (Courtesy of Nuclear Associates, Carle Place, NY.)

phantom with linear resolution capabilities should also be available, as should a set of T1 and T2 standards (Figure 11–3). These T1 and T2 solutions should cover the range of physiologic values observed in several steps (six to twelve). These solutions can be purchased or a very stable set of standards can be made from progressive dilutions of propylene glycol (10% steps) in deionized water. These "home-made" standards contain both water and organic protons, and the relaxation times are the average of the mixture.

The uniformity phantom should be imaged the first thing each morning, and the tip angles and center frequencies should be recorded. The phantom should then be imaged with a standard sequence that is closely related to the type of imaging most commonly done on the system. The uniformity of the slices should be examined and the signal-to-noise ratio should be calculated for the center slice; the value should be recorded

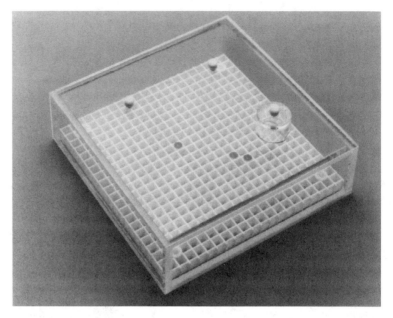

Figure 11–2. Uniformity and linearity phantom. (Courtesy of Nuclear Associates, Carle Place, NY.)

in a log book. Someone should be assigned the responsibility of checking these values weekly, looking for trends that indicate that the system is moving away from baseline values.

Relaxation times of the standards can be arranged around the phantoms, and they should be measured at least weekly to ensure that proper changes in tissue contrast are obtained while scanning. Basic magnet performance is assured if uniformity, reproducibility, and T1 and T2 contrast can be maintained. Additional parameters can be checked using phantoms or by electronic means. Electronic techniques usually require the services of a physicist or field service engineer, as the methodology and interpretation can become complex. Slice and gap thicknesses can be measured by simple integral methods (slice profile or signals ratio). Spatial linearity and resolution inserts can be included in the uniformity phantom, although specialized phantoms that allow testing over wide ranges are also available (Figure 11–4). Oblique projections can

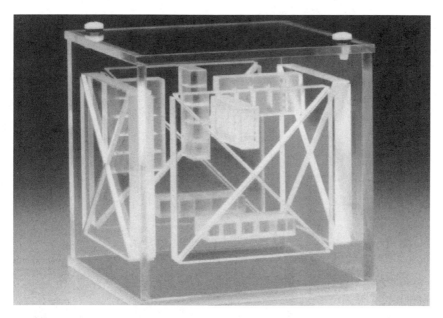

Figure 11–3.   Slice thickness, high-contrast resolution phantom. (Courtesy of Nuclear Associates, Carle Place, NY.)

be examined. Exotic pulse sequences and data-acquisition strategies can be used and electronic measurements made.

Experience may indicate that some of these other parameters rarely change, provided that certain basic parameters (tip angles, uniformity, SNR, and phantom shape) have not changed. Once MRI personnel obtain this experience, they do not need to undertake more complicated procedures as frequently. It is the learning process that customizes QA procedures to the most cost-effective form for a particular piece of equipment. Of course, if an anomaly is detected, more elaborate and specific tests should be performed.

QA is almost completely dependent upon systematic and comprehensive recordkeeping. Special forms have been used for MRI and other areas of diagnostic radiology, but a hard-backed notebook without loose pages offers significant advantages. The notebook approach tends to control potential loss of data kept on pieces of paper, which can often be misplaced or

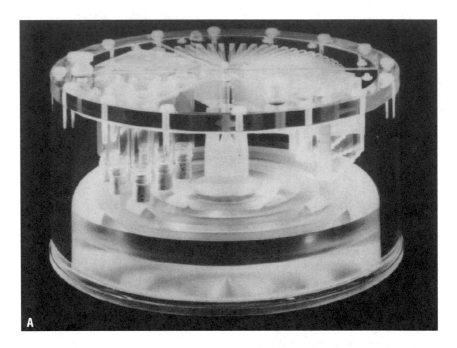

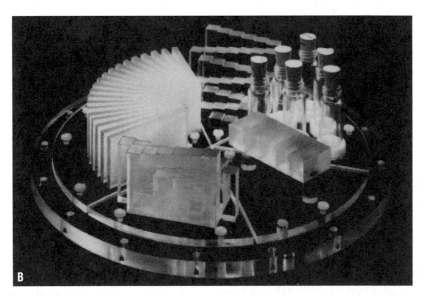

Figure 11–4. Multipurpose phantom provides multiple interchangeable components (A and B) for a comprehensive range of tests for slice thickness, spatial resolution, rf signal uniformity, magnetic field homogeneity, and T1 and T2 evaluations. (Courtesy of Nuclear Associates, Carle Place, NY.)

lost. The raw data as well as any calculations should be recorded in all cases. QA records are often more significant in retrospect than was evident at the time of the recording. If a computer terminal is near the operating console, setting up a database or spreadsheet program offers distinct advantages. Computer searches, correlations, and graphing can be done almost instantaneously, and this may ultimately be the most efficient form of recordkeeping.

ARCHIVING

Computer components are steadily becoming more sophisticated, and disk storage capacity continues to increase. Unfortunately, disk capacity on a system is usually fixed when the system is installed. This fixed disk space, whether on a single disk or on multiple disks, must be allocated for software among MR operations, software for reconstruction, raw data, and image data. Software requirements are initially established at a defined quantity, but with changes and upgrades, software often requires an increasingly larger portion of the available disk space. The growth of this requirement usually is not noticeable, but it can be appreciable with major system upgrades. If storage problems are observed, larger disk capacity should be requested from the manufacturer.

Raw data and image data consume extremely large amounts of storage space. Older units may still require a manual deletion of raw data, but most systems will automatically delete the raw data soon after images are reconstructed. The rapid and automated data removal keeps procedures flowing smoothly, keeps disks relatively uncluttered, and prevents a slowdown in procedures due to limited disk space. With the increased usage of three-dimensional imaging and vascular imaging, both of which require large amounts of disk space, free disk space is again becoming a problem. It is possible for the available free space to become so fragmented that contiguous free space is inadequate even though there is adequate total free space. Loss of contiguous free space can degrade performance or produce errors in software execution. These errors are often intermittent, making detection more difficult. An analysis of the configuration of system disks and storage disks should be undertaken if performance errors are not corrected by other means.

The problem with rapid data removal is that once removed it is no longer available for image reconstruction. If a reconstruction error occurred and wasn't noticed, or if images were deleted before they were archived, the entire study is lost and cannot be retrieved. It is good practice (1) to check images immediately for proper reconstruction; and (2) to archive data as soon as possible. Images should be checked as they are being reconstructed, not only for reconstruction errors but for positioning and image quality as well. Patients should remain in the examination area until personnel can confirm the quality of all of the images. On occasion some of the later images are not reconstructed, so all images should be checked before the patient leaves.

Images should be archived as soon as possible so that they are not accidentally erased and so that they can be deleted to open more space on the disk. Different centers handle image archival and retention of studies quite differently. Images can be stored on magnetic tape or on optical disks. Magnetic tape is much cheaper, is reusable, and no longer requires significant storage space. The large 12-inch reel-to-reel tapes have been replaced by 8-mm DAT tapes, which are smaller than an audio cassette. The 12-inch reels were able to hold 211 256-by-256 images, while the DAT tapes can hold over 14,000 such images, or over 4,500 512-by-512 images. Optical disks are much more expensive but are quicker and more permanent than magnetic tape. The policies of individual MRI centers, which may be affected by state law, vary significantly.

At Cornell, our policy has been to store images permanently, so we archive all images on optical disks. Formerly, some sites would archive images on magnetic tape and delete them after a few weeks, reusing the tape as they did so. These images were kept just long enough to make sure that the photography was adequate and then held for a short while in case additional copies were requested. The cost of 12-inch reels and the additional cost of storage space were significant factors for some in deciding not to archive studies permanently. This rationale is no longer valid, as the 8-mm DAT tapes cost less than $3 apiece, hold many images, and require very little in the way of storage space. Currently, there does not appear to be any reason not to archive studies permanently: the decision to be made is whether to utilize magnetic tape or optical disk.

Optical disks are sturdier, withstand more handling, restore images much more rapidly, and can withstand a wider range of temperature and humidity than can magnetic tapes. Storage is no longer a factor for either media. On the downside, the cost per study with optical disks is significantly higher, with each 5.5-inch disk, capable of holding 4,000 256-by-256 images or 1,000 512-by-512 images, costing approximately $100.

Magnetic tapes must be kept out of a magnetic environment. The current recommendation of 10 G as a maximum safe level for magnetic tapes was formulated for analog tapes with an expected life of 20 to 30 years. This is a very conservative limit for digital tapes since the discontinuous signal levels of the digital format is much less sensitive to small background changes than the continuous nature of analog signals. Magnetic materials used in tapes typically undergo transition between 200 and 300 G, so a limit of 50 G appears sufficient for short-term storage and probably is also adequate for long-term storage. Degradation of magnetic tape is more commonly caused by heat and humidity than by magnetic fields. For long-term storage, tapes should be stored in a relatively low-humidity area in which extremes of temperature are avoided.

A critical problem can arise from tape-head adjustments. If the tape heads become adjusted incorrectly, it is possible that tapes can be recorded and read, but old tapes that were recorded under the old adjustment will be indecipherable. To prevent this, personnel should check the unit weekly either by reading a standardized tape or, equivalently, by reading an old tape.

A seemingly obvious but essential aspect of archival storage is the proper labeling and cataloging of all archived studies, whether on tape or on disk. Without the proper records to locate a given study rapidly, the best-kept archives are of limited use. This database can be maintained electronically or conventionally in logbooks or file cards. At a minimum, the record should contain the patient's name, identification number, type of study, and tape or disk number. If there is the possibility of using the studies for research, it would be advantageous to include additional data (diagnosis, findings, etc.).

In summary, a practical QA program for archival includes periodic testing of tape heads, inspecting to be sure that tape is stored under proper conditions, and assuring that personnel are properly labeling and recording the studies.

PHOTOGRAPHY

Photographic tastes and techniques vary for different types of examinations and different individuals. For example, some radiologists prefer high-contrast magnified images to evaluate the knee for meniscal tears. Photographic technique is especially important in MRI since changes in contrast on the different pulse sequences are utilized to make a diagnosis. Practice and experience, along with a knowledge of what type of diagnostic information is being sought, are the most important factors in proper photography. Constructive criticism by the radiologist is necessary in order to master appropriate technique.

The obvious goal in photographing a study is to reproduce on film the exact image presented on the display screen. While this seems a simple task, it can prove to be surprisingly difficult. Both the display and the camera (regular or laser multiformat camera) must be adjusted in synch so that what the operator sees on the screen is what comes out on the film. The appearance of the film depends upon the performance of the multiformatter, which is affected by the screen brightness, contrast, and density; film processing conditions; viewbox brightness; background lighting levels; and viewing distance. Display screens permit brightness and contrast levels to be set. Electronically, the brightness represents a base level and the contrast is a gain. The brightness sets the level of the darkest parts of the image, and the contrast determines how quickly the transition between dark to light occurs. The display screen must be adjusted before the camera can be tuned.

The multiformat camera has an exposure time adjustment, which is called the **density adjustment**, in addition to the brightness and contrast controls. When the display is fixed, the camera adjustments are varied until the image on film matches the image on the screen. The values of the contrast, brightness, and density should be recorded if needed in the future. Increasing the brightness will darken the image significantly, increase the contrast between light objects, and decrease the contrast between dark objects; increasing the contrast will darken the image slightly, will not change the contrast between light objects, and will significantly decrease the contrast between dark objects; increasing the density will darken the image moderately, increase the contrast between the bright objects, and virtually eliminate contrast between dark objects. The use of a test pattern is invaluable in determining proper settings for the camera (Figure 11–5). The type of film is also critical in selecting accurate values for the camera. If the type of film is changed, the entire calibration procedure must be repeated.

Film-processing conditions are the most significant remaining variable. Often problems in the appearance of images are due to problems with the film processor (improper chemical mix, dirty rollers, temperature fluctuations), and a regular preventative maintenance program should be strictly followed. Gradual changes in the quality of images is very difficult to perceive, especially if the evaluator is looking at films every day. For this reason, a good QA program should include a monthly comparison of films of studies performed over large periods of time (e.g., a study from today should be compared with one from a month ago, and one from six months ago, and one from a year ago, etc.).

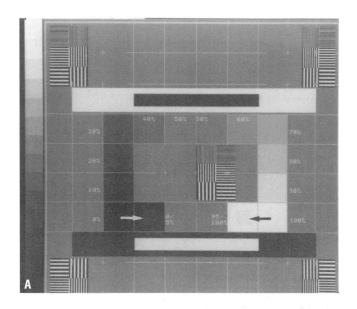

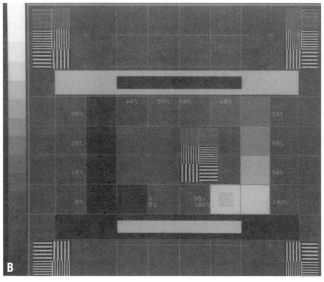

Figure 11–5. (A) Normal test pattern from a multiformat camera. Each box of the gray scale is numbered as a percentage of gray scale, from 0% to 100%. In addition, two boxes (arrows) allow differentiation of signal at the bright and dark ends of the spectrum. The 100–95% box represents contrast at the bright end (black arrow), while the 0–5% box represents contrast at the dark end (white arrow). (B) Increasing the brightness substantially darkens the image, increases the 100–95% contrast, and decreases the 0–5% contrast.

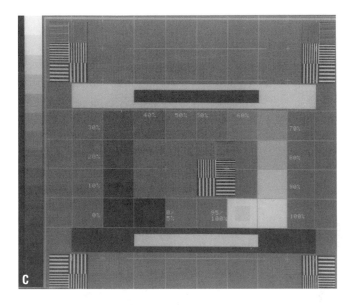

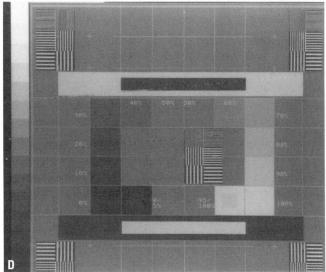

Figure 11–5. *(cont.)*   (C) Increasing the contrast darkens the image slightly, leaves the 100–95% contrast unchanged, and eliminates the 0–5% contrast. (D) Increasing the density darkens the image, increases the 100–95% contrast, and eliminates the distinction between 0% and 10%.

POINTS TO PONDER

- QA programs should be designed so that they provide clues to solving a problem as soon as it occurs, or preferably, to predict a failure that can be corrected before it happens.

- Efficient QA programs are based on careful observations of performance over time.

- A uniformity phantom is necessary for any QA program.

- Phantoms should be of such size that they almost completely fill the field of view. Thus at least two phantoms are required: one for the head coil and one for the body coil.

- A set of T1 and T2 standards should be imaged periodically.

- Effective QA is dependent upon accurate, routine, and comprehensive record-keeping.

- Loss of contiguous free space on a system disk can result in poor performance and/or produce errors in software execution.

- Images should be checked before a patient is allowed to leave.

- Images should be archived as soon as possible.

- Heat and humidity are more of a threat to successful storage of magnetic tapes than magnetic fields.

- Tape heads should be periodically tested.

- Image quality should be routinely tested and compared to older studies.

CHAPTER TWELVE

PATIENTS REQUIRE PATIENCE

The ultimate goal of any diagnostic procedure is to determine the cause of the patient's problem so that a cure can be effected. In addition, because the examination is relatively long and patients often have to wait for appointments, procedures must be adjusted to be of high diagnostic quality, while still maximizing the total number of studies completed. The reactions of individual patients to impending MRI studies are quite varied and pose a wide range of problems that put completion of the examination at risk. Dealing with these problems and helping the patients to cope with their anxiety is essential to enable successful completion of the study.

It must always be kept in mind that any patient undergoing an MRI procedure is suffering from symptoms of one type or another, or has a known medical condition and is being further evaluated. Any patient undergoing an MRI will, almost by definition, be anxious. It is incumbent upon the entire staff of the imaging center—physicians, technologists, nurses, and secretarial staff—to understand the potential stress that the patient and his or her family is under, and to try all available means to relieve their anxiety, make their experience comfortable, and be as supportive as possible.

A large part of this, of course, is personal interaction. Closely coupled to this is the operation of an efficient, well-planned program that will make the patients feel at ease and allow them to realize that they are in the hands of a competent and professional organization. Appearances and personal interactions are key to making the patient feel confident, and this begins with the initial phone call to confirm the patient's appointment.

All patients can be divided into two broad categories: in-patients and out-patients. An in-patient is defined as someone who has been admitted to a hospital; an out-patient is someone who is coming in for the examination from home. Hospital-based MRI units will encounter both types of patients while facilities not connected directly to a hospital will rarely image an in-patient. Hospitalized patients require extra screening because they are usually ill or recuperating and may have IV setups, IV pumps, respirators, monitors, and other equipment not normally associated with the out-patient population. In almost all other ways, all patients should be treated in a similar manner.

Patient screening and preparation should start on the hospital floor for in-patients, in the clinic, or at the referring physician's office. Referring physicians, nurses, secretaries, and clerks should be made aware of the potentials and limitations of MRI so that the screening process can begin as early as possible. In this way patients with cardiac pacemakers and magnetic cerebral aneurysm clips could be eliminated very early in the scheduling process. If the patient has metallic implants or prostheses, all involved personnel should be sufficiently aware of potential problems so that they question the MRI receptionist, radiologist, or technologist to determine if such items might interfere with the examination or pose a potential hazard to the patient. They should also be made aware of the current guidelines about pregnant patients, so that they can make an intelligent decision whether the scan should be scheduled, and will be able to discuss the situation with the patient.

To achieve this increased awareness among referring personnel, and to disseminate this knowledge to patients, the distribution of pamphlets is quite helpful. These brochures should explain the general nature of the MRI exam, the type of equipment used, the time required for studies, and all conditions that would exclude the patient from being a candidate for an examination (see Table 9–4). It is extremely important to explain the nature of the "tunnel" in which the patient lies during the procedure so that patients who are slightly anxious can express their fears openly before the examination, and proper steps can be taken to reassure them before the examination. Since 1983, we have scanned over 80,000 patients; fewer than 0.5% have refused studies because of claustrophobia or anxiety. With the proper handling of patients, beginning with the initial phone call, almost all patients can undergo an MRI study.

INITIAL PATIENT INTERACTION

When the appointment is made, the receptionist must obtain the correct spelling of the patient's name; telephone numbers at which the patient can be reached; the name, address, telephone, and fax number of the physician; the precise type of study that is being requested (routine head, head with pituitary views, head with optic nerve views, with or without contrast, etc.); and a diagnosis relating to the reason that the patient is having the scan. Patients very often have more than one condition, and a physician's secretary may read a diagnosis from a patient's chart that is not at all related to his or her current problem (e.g., hypertension for a knee study).

After the appointment is made by the physician's office, for out-patients a telephone call is made two to three days in advance of the scheduled study. During this phone call, the receptionist will confirm the date and time of the appointment with the patient, inform the patient of the address of the facility, tells the patient what to bring (e.g., insurance forms, workman's compensation authorization, etc.), verify insurance information, and either answer any questions that the patient may have or transfer the call to a technologist or radiologist to answer the questions. The patient should also be told to eat normally and that all medications should be taken as usual. During this call the patient screening process continues, as the patient should be questioned about pacemakers, cerebral aneurysm clips, pregnancy, or other conditions that might affect the patient's qualification as a candidate for the exam. With the increasing role of HMOs in medicine, obtaining precertification has become necessary with some health care providers, so that obtaining accurate information from the patient is essential.

ARRIVING AT THE MR SUITE

After arriving at the MRI facility, the patient is usually interviewed by four persons: a receptionist, a billing clerk, a technologist, and a physician. Each has his or her own special interests, but each also should enforce certain basic themes: cardiac pacemakers are not allowed; the patient must lie motionless during the study; the examination is not as difficult as the patient may have heard; someone can come into the scanning room with the patient. Each of these interviewers should be familiar with the types of patients who cannot have scans, and each should check to be sure.

The receptionist greets the patient and verifies the patient's identity and demographic information. An in-patient's I.D. band and patient chart should be checked as well. The patient is asked to fill out a short questionnaire designed to eliminate possible complications and to make the radiologist aware of surgical hardware, prior surgery, and other pertinent medical history. The receptionist is responsible for knowing exactly which patients have arrived, which patients are waiting in the waiting area, and which have gone in for scans.

The billing clerk is primarily interested in billing details and insurance forms. The proper ICD9 code for the study must be determined and insurance information verified. The seemingly unlimited variations in health care policies are usually quite confusing to the patient, and the billing clerk has the responsibility of ascertaining the particulars to aid the patient in understanding his or her obligations. The billing clerk must also determine that precertification, when necessary, has been obtained in advance of the patient's arrival.

The radiologist checks the gathered information to ensure that there will be no complications from any surgical implant or foreign body and that the correct region of the body will be imaged with the most appropriate sequences. The radiologist should determine the imaging sequence protocol and may want to consult by telephone with the referring physician to check on the medical details. The radiologist should reassure the patient and answer any questions.

MEETING THE TECHNOLOGIST

The technologist is ultimately responsible for the safety of the patient and for performing a proper examination. She or he is the final check to confirm that the patient does not have any of the contraindications for being examined. At the same time the patient must be reassured that there is no hazard associated with hip replacements, CSF shunts, sternal sutures, and other known safe surgical devices. Notes should be made to the radiologist of any implants or surgery, to aid in interpreting the study. Metal detectors can be useful for resolving questions about the presence of metallic articles. The use of a portable, hand-held metal detector to determine the presence of internal metallic devices is used in some centers, thought to be unnecessary in others, but certainly does have its merits. Sometimes even the most thorough questioning is not enough. Hand-held models may not be sensitive enough to detect small internal metal objects, however, and the degree of localization is questionable (e.g., dental prostheses can produce significant readings in the area of the eye). However, although they many not be able to detect magnetic aneurysm clips or ocular foreign bodies, metal detectors will detect pacemakers, guns (police officers are quite reluctant to part with their weapons when undergoing a scan), and loose magnetic objects.

In addition, the technologist must determine the anxiety level of the patient and assess how much assistance will be needed in handling him or her. The technologist should tell the patient approximately how long the examination should be, and also impress on the patient the importance of remaining still during the data-acquisition sequences; in addition, unless it is contraindicated (e.g., if the pelvis is being examined), the technologist should encourage the patient to use the bathroom facilities. The patient should be reassured that the examination is safe and painless and will provide the referring physician with diagnostic information that will help in his or her medical treatment.

Patients arriving in wheelchairs or on stretchers should be handled very conservatively. A technologist should not attempt to transfer a debilitated patient onto the imaging table alone. Assistance should always be sought in such cases. Since some stretchers and wheelchairs can be attracted to the magnet, it is safer to undock the imaging table and transfer these patients onto the table outside of the imaging room. Care should be taken with in-patients, making sure that IV poles are not magnetic and that no metallic devices, clips, or staples are present.

Prior to scanning, the technologist must complete and reinforce the educational process that started when the patient was first scheduled and has been advanced through the various interviews. Patients who are having head or cervical spine studies do not have to be gowned and can go into the magnet dressed in their clothes. The patient should be instructed to remove metal hair clips or hair pins, and to remove any jewelry and watches as well. Although gold should not produce an artifact on the scan, very often clips on gold earrings and catches on bracelets are not made of gold and can produce very large artifacts. For this reason we suggest that all jewelry be removed. The burden of watching a patient's jewelry should not be placed upon the technologist, and every facility should provide lockers for the patients' valuables—not only objects but also wallets, purses, and so on. If a patient is being gowned for a study below the neck, individual removal of the items is not necessary, as it will all be left in the locker with the patient's clothing. The patient is now ready to enter the scanning room.

The procedure should again be explained. Points that should be stressed by the technologist include:

- The importance of lying still during the procedure.
- The noise and movement of the table should be mentioned, so that there are no surprises from sudden table motion.
- Ear plugs should be provided at this time.
- The patient should be reassured that there is a microphone in the bore of the magnet so that the technologist can hear anything said by the patient.
- There are also a set of speakers so that the technologist can be heard by the patient.

Before beginning the scanning process it is always a good idea to test the microphone and speakers in order to provide additional reassurance to the patient.

The patient is now ready to begin the actual scanning process. One cardinal rule is that a patient should always be attended by someone when in the imaging room, except while being scanned. The patient should be helped onto the imaging table. Although the tables can be lowered, very often they do not go down quite far enough to permit easy access to elderly or disabled patients. A small one-step wooden platform will make entry and exit a much easier process for all patients. Assistance should be provided as the patient first sits, then lies down on the table. Many patients are unsteady, and someone should be present and prepared to prevent a mishap.

It is important that the patient be positioned comfortably on the table. Patients are much more likely to remain motionless during the exam if they are comfortably positioned on the table from the beginning; motion-degraded images and the necessity to have sequences repeated can thus be reduced. If they are not being imaged in the head coil, they should have their head placed on a pillow. A wedge-shaped pillow placed beneath the patients' knees not only makes them more comfortable, but also relieves pressure on their backs; this is especially important in patients being imaged for back pain. Pediatric patients should be raised up on blankets or other support, to get them closer to the axis of the magnet, where the homogeneity of the magnetic field is best and better images will be obtained. Surface coils should be accurately positioned with respect to the region to be imaged and should be properly secured to prevent their moving. Restraining straps are usually available for the head and other parts of the body, which help to position the patient properly and serve as a reminder not to move; however, the use of these restrictions will often add to a patient's anxiety and can do more harm than good.

THE "CLAUSTROPHOBIC" PATIENT

Our experience has been that there are actually very few truly claustrophobic patients, and that most patients can complete the examination if a few potential problems are anticipated. Less than 0.5% of our patients fail to complete the examination, which is significantly less than reported at many other centers. The technologist must realize that some things that we take for granted can be anxiety-provoking or even frightening to someone who has never experienced it before. The patient arriving at the scanning room is nervous for a variety of reasons as outlined above. Additionally, MRI has received "bad press" with many people playing up the claustrophobic aspect of the scanning procedure. Entering the bore of the magnet for the first time is not the most pleasant of sensations; however, if MRI personnel downplay the experience, patients will not anticipate a problem.

A true claustrophobic, one who has a fear of confined spaces, is not a candidate for an MRI examination unless he or she is sedated. These patients cannot ride in elevators or enter small rooms (closets) and often have problems with airplanes. Most people are somewhat uncomfortable in confined spaces, although they have no problem coping with them for short periods of time. The majority of patients fall into the latter category; however, if they are convinced that there is a severe problem with being confined in the magnet, this concern coupled with their worries about their health and what may be found during the examination may increase their anxiety levels to a point that prevents them from completing the examination. Several steps can be taken to educate the patient and alleviate their fears and anxieties, and to increase the likelihood of a completed test.

Referring physicians and their staffs, particularly secretaries who make the appointments, should be made aware that the magnet is not as confining as is sometimes thought, and that there are several ways that the anxious patient can be calmed. The suggestion of a claustrophobic reaction can provoke an anxiety attack, which would not have occurred without the allusion to the possibility. During the confirmation process, the MRI secretary should never ask the patient if he or she is claustrophobic. If the question of claustrophobia arises, the patient should be asked if he or she is truly claustrophobic (for example, can the patient not ride in elevators?). If the patient is just anxious, the secretary should offer reassuring information:

- The study is relatively easy.
- The magnet is open at both ends.
- The information will help the physician obtain a diagnosis, or to further evaluate the patient's condition.
- The examination is noninvasive, has no ionizing radiation, and may render unnecessary a much more invasive procedure, such as angiography or laparoscopy.
- Someone can accompany the patient into the magnet room during the examination.
- The patient is in constant contact with the technologist by a microphone and speaker.
- The patient can be taken out immediately at any time during the examination if there is a problem.
- If feeling uncomfortable, the patient can be moved out of the magnet after each sequence, allowing time to rest and gain composure.

If the patient still has doubts, he or she should be invited to the facility in advance of the appointment to "visit" the MRI system and observe exactly what is going to happen. It is usually the fear of the unknown that is most frightening, and observing what will happen during the procedure is almost always enough to reassure the patient that there will not be a problem. In extreme cases, a mild tranquilizer can be prescribed, although in our experience this is necessary in less than one in 500 cases.

Patient education at the facility begins with a friendly greeting by the receptionist. Patient information brochures should be available, and sometimes a video cassette demonstrating the procedure can be shown in the waiting room. If a patient arrives alone and is still anxious when arriving at the scanning room, a technologist can stay in the room, providing encouragement and assurance that assistance is only steps away. A friend or relative can provide the same service and is probably more reassuring. Usually closing the eyes is sufficient to allay the worries of a patient who is only slightly apprehensive. Using a combination of these techniques, most patients are able to comfortably complete the examination.

Several different devices have been proposed to allay patient fears and to distract them while entering the magnet. The patient can wear periscope-type glasses so that he or she can see out through the front of the bore. Glasses with a permanent picture have been employed to let the patient's eyes rest upon a pleasant scene. Audio systems are available that do not interfere with the rf signal of the study and permit the patient to listen to music of his or her choice. There are even MR-compatible video systems available to entertain the patient with a videotape (Figure 12–1). Although none of these embellishments is absolutely necessary for a successful examination, they can go a long way, when available, toward convincing patients that they will not be bothered by the confining aspects of the system.

The technologist should always be pleasant, encouraging and eager to answer any questions that the patient might have. The patient should NEVER be rushed onto the imaging table. If the patient is nervous, an experienced technologist may sense

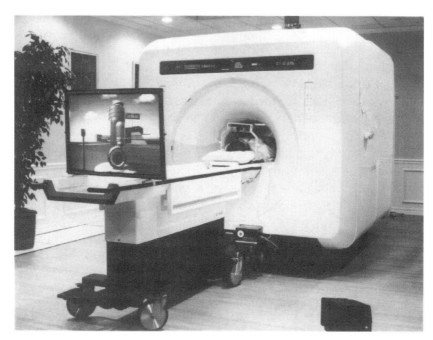

Figure 12–1. HI-TECH MRI Video System for entertaining patients while they are being scanned. A reflection mirror allows the patient to remain supine and view the TV screen from inside the bore. (Courtesy of Nuclear Associates, Carle Place, NY.)

that there is a danger of an incomplete examination. He or she can take any of the following steps to reassure the patient and shorten the time of the study, in addition to the ones mentioned on the previous page:

- Modify the imaging protocol to shorten imaging time.
- Obtain the most important sequences first—an incomplete protocol may still be diagnostic.
- Use fast spin-echo techniques.
- Place the patient prone, if practical, so that he or she can see out.
- Remain in communication with the patient in between sequences via the speakers.
- Physically enter the imaging room at the end of each sequence to speak to the patient in person, until the patient is comfortable.

PRACTICAL IMAGING TIPS

Shortening the imaging time while maintaining a high-quality study is important not only for the anxious patient but also for the patient in medical distress. It is also useful when additional emergency patients are added to the schedule, unanticipated patient problems cause delays, patients arrive late, and system failures occur. As noted in previous chapters, several variables can control the imaging time of a single sequence, and each has different effects on the resolution of the images obtained (Table 12–1). The easiest way to decrease imaging time can be applied to all studies, and that is to eliminate what we consider a "useless" sequence. Many protocols call for an initial scout series, employing a fast imaging sequence with thick sections. This low-contrast study is of very limited, if any, diagnostic value. Even though imaging time is often less than one minute, actual room utilization time is considerably more when tuning is considered. It is much more effective if the patient is landmarked properly and a useful diagnostic series is directly obtained as the initial series. These images can then be used to prescribe further series. A T1-weighted series will add approximately one minute to the total "scout" imaging time, but will provide relevant diagnostic information. This "useful scout" series can be applied in any type of study.

TABLE 12–1. EFFECT OF CHANGING SCANNING PARAMETERS ON IMAGING TIME AND IMAGE APPEARANCE

Parameter	Change	Imaging Time	Image Appearance
Repetition time	Decrease	Decreases	Image contrast changed
N_{ex}	Decrease	Decreases	SNR decreases
Matrix	Decrease	Decreases	Resolution decreases
Number of slices	Decrease	Decreases[1]	No change[2]
FOV	Decrease	None[3]	Increased resolution; decreased SNR
Fractional FOV	Decrease	Decreases	No change
Spin-echo	Use FSE	Decreases	Some contrast decrease
Bandwidth	Increase	Decreases	SNR and resolution decrease

1. Imaging time will decrease only if more than one acquisition has been prescribed.
2. Image contrast, resolution, and SNR remain unchanged.
3. The number of available slices may decrease if FOV is made too small, thereby increasing imaging time by requiring additional acquisitions.

The basic equation for determining imaging time is

Imaging time =
(repetition time) × (number of phase-encoding steps)
× (number of excitations) / 1,000

Using abbreviations, it can be rewritten as

$$\textbf{Time} = \textbf{TR} \times N_p \times N_{ex} / \textbf{1,000}$$

The repetition time, TR, can be shortened and will directly decrease the imaging time. This is not, however, a valid method of saving time during a scan because shortening the imaging time will also affect other variables; most notably, it will decrease the relative contrast of the tissues. By shortening the repetition time, the relative T2 weighting of the images is decreased and the appearance of the image will be significantly altered (Figure 12–2).

The second term in the time equation is the number of phase-encoding steps, which is the matrix size in the phase-encoding direction. This can vary, usually in increments of 64 steps, from 128 to 512. As previously mentioned, the higher the value, the greater the resolution. Each pixel is smaller as the matrix is increased, so that smaller structures can be distinguished. SNR, however, decreases since the amount of signal in each pixel (or voxel) is smaller because of the smaller size. If a

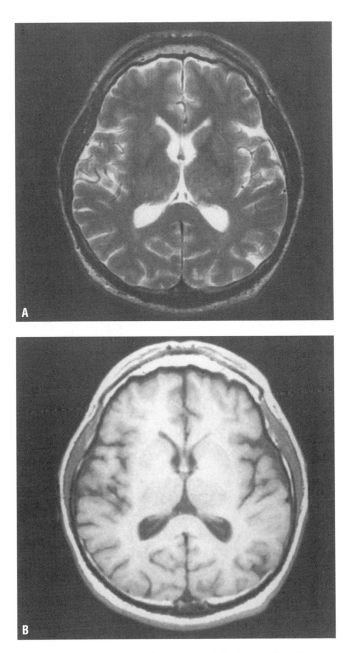

Figure 12–2.   (A) T2-weighted axial image of the head. (B) The same image as in A, but the TR has been reduced to obtain a T1-weighted image. Notice the lack of contrast between the structures when compared to A.

patient is having a problem with the scan, the matrix size can usually be decreased slightly without a significant loss in diagnostic ability (Figure 12–3). Decreasing the matrix from 256 to 192, for example, will increase pixel size for a head study (24-cm FOV) from 0.94 mm to 1.25 mm, while shortening the time of the sequence by 25%. This slight decrease in resolution is usually better than not completing the examination, or than having the patient move during the longer acquisition time, thereby significantly decreasing resolution.

The last term in the time equation is the number of excitations, or number of signal averages. In principle, the greater the N_{ex}, the higher the SNR and the less grainy and more pleasing the image. The increase in SNR, however, is only as the square root of the N_{ex}, whereas the increase in time is directly proportional. Doubling the N_{ex} will double the time of the study, but it will increase the SNR only by the square root of 2, or 41%. Attempts to provide better images by increasing the N_{ex} will sometimes backfire, since lengthening the acquisition time too much will increase the chances that the patient will move. When imaging time has to be decreased, decreasing the N_{ex} is an acceptable way to achieve it. Changing from 2 N_{ex} to 1 N_{ex} will cut the imaging time in half but decrease the SNR by only 29%. This is most acceptable in a coil with an inherently high signal and low noise, such as the head coil. Figure 12–4 demonstrates the effect of decreasing the N_{ex} on the quality of the image.

Although only three terms in the equation determine the total imaging time, there are other methods to accomplish shorter scans. Occasionally too many slices are prescribed for a given study. A given spin-echo sequence at TR of 500 ms (0.5 seconds) will permit acquisition of 15 slices at an imaging time of 2 minutes and 8 seconds. If 18 seconds are prescribed, two acquisitions must be obtained and the imaging time increases to 4 minutes and 16 seconds. If the number of slices is cut back to 15, only the area of interest is covered, and imaging time will be 2 minutes and 8 seconds. For T2-weighted acquisitions this can increase from 11 minutes to 22 minutes if too many slices are requested.

The bandwidth is the range of frequencies that a given voxel will interact with. A wide bandwidth includes more noise with the true signal than does a narrow bandwidth, which will

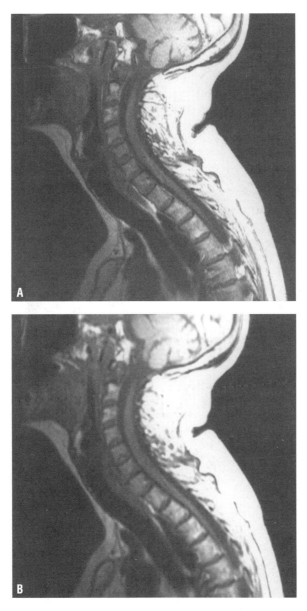

Figure 12–3. (A) Sagittal image of the cervical spine obtained with a 512-by-192 matrix. (B) Same section as in A, but with the matrix decreased to 256-by-128. Resolution in A is much higher than in B, as can be observed by the sharper definition of structures such as the vertebral bodies and cerebellum in A and relative blurring in B. SNR is higher in B because voxel size is larger and contains more signal, so that image A is grainier. Total imaging time saved was just over 1 minute.

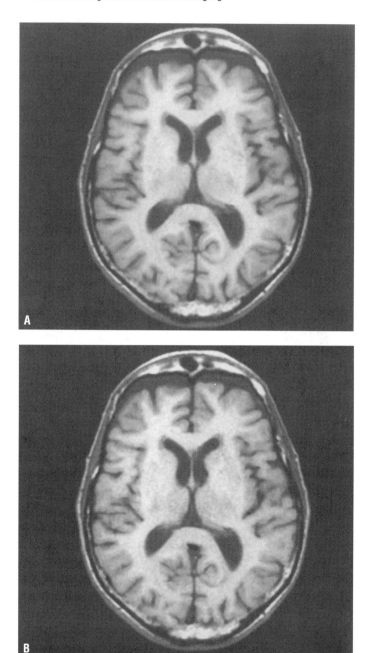

Figure 12–4.   (A) Axial image of the head obtained at 2 N_{ex}. (B) Same section as in A, but with the N_{ex} decreased to 1. Note that image B is slightly noisier, but resolution is not significantly affected.

reduce the noise collected by the receiver. A narrow bandwidth would appear to be preferable, but the sampling time is related to the bandwidth. If the bandwidth is decreased too much, the scanning time and the TE will have to be increased. Increasing the bandwidth will permit a smaller TE, increase the number of slices available, and decrease imaging time.

In the right situations a fractional FOV will decrease imaging time by 25% to 50% (Figures 8–25 and 8–26). This method will work only if the entire image does not fill the field of view and, as noted in Chapter 8, the section of the image not sampled is in the direction of the phase-encoding gradient.

Imaging time can be significantly decreased by the use of fast spin-echo (FSE) pulse sequences instead of the regular spin-echo acquisitions (Chapter 6). Imaging times can be decreased by factors of 8, 16, or more when using FSE techniques. There are two trade-offs to using FSE: image contrast is not quite as high as with regular spin echo, and the number of available slices is decreased. For T1-weighted images this does not significantly change the overall imaging time, since the number of slices decreases and multiple acquisitions must be used. For example, using a TR of 500 ms, a spin-echo technique that requires 15 slices would take 2 minutes and 28 seconds. Eighteen slices would be allowed in a single acquisition. The same FSE technique would permit only 3 slices per acquisition but would take only 12 seconds. Five acquisitions, therefore, would be necessary to obtain all 15 slices, and the total imaging time would be 1 minute and 41 seconds. The saving of 47 seconds is relatively trivial. The only advantage would be for patients who cannot lie still, since each 12-second acquisition would be reconstructed separately. If a patient did not move for those 12 seconds, the images would be perfect. The only images that would be blurred would be those obtained in any 12-second interval during which the patient moved. In this way not all the images would be blurred by motion artifact, as would be the case during a regular spin-echo sequence.

The big savings in time with FSE sequences is during long TR images (T2-weighted acquisitions). For example, a regular spin-echo sequence with a TR of 3,000 ms (3.0 seconds) and echo times of 17 ms and 102 ms would permit acquisition of 29 slices in 14 minutes and 36 seconds. The same FSE sequence, with an echo train of 8 (8 simultaneous acquisitions), would only permit 19 slices but would decrease the imaging time to 3 minutes and 48 seconds, a savings of almost 11 minutes in imaging time. In order to compensate for the decreased contrast, in this particular case, a TR of 4,000 ms might be used to increase the T2 weighting, which would increase imaging time to almost 5 minutes, resulting in a 9-minute decrease in imaging time. Unfortunately, FSE is not compatible with respiratory compensation techniques necessary to eliminate artifacts in the chest and abdomen.

Protocols are useful time savers. With current computer power decreasing reconstruction time and permitting sequences to be prescribed in advance, it is actually quicker to do an additional series rather than wait for the images to be reviewed by the radiologist, who then would decide to whether or not an additional sequence is necessary. In our experience, by the time the decision is made, the additional sequence would have been completed. Protocols for all of our studies are prepared in advance. Although we have standard protocols (e.g., routine head, pituitary, IAC, post-op LS spine, female pelvis), the pulse sequences for each study are decided in advance by the radiologists, individualized to the patient's diagnosis and particular medical problem. Additional sequences can be added, if necessary, as the images are reconstructed. The individualized protocols, however, are usually sufficient to provide adequate diagnostic information. Technologists, especially experienced ones, will often observe an unsuspected abnormality and bring it to the attention of a radiologist. When additional sequences are necessary they should be performed, since there are no harmful effects to the patient and the patient will not have to return for additional views.

POINTS TO PONDER

- Patients require patience.

- Patient education is of prime importance in securing patient confidence and a proper scan.

- Patient education begins with referring physicians and their staff.

- Patient reassurance and education are the responsibility of the entire MRI staff.

- Metal detectors can be useful for detecting unsuspected metallic objects.

- Nervous or anxious patients should be treated very gently.

- Most patients are not really claustrophobic and can successfully be scanned if given some extra attention from the entire staff.

- Ear plugs should be provided to all patients.

- For nervous patients, imaging protocols can be modified so that imaging time is shortened.

- Total imaging time of a given spin-echo sequence (in seconds) is equal to the product of the repetition time, the number of phase-encoding steps, and the number of excitations (signal averages) divided by 1,000.

- Imaging time can be shortened (without significantly decreasing diagnostic accuracy) by decreasing N_{ex}, by decreasing the number of phase-encoding steps, by increasing the bandwidth, by using a fractional FOV, or by using fast imaging techniques.

- Using fast spin-echo sequences is the most acceptable method of decreasing imaging time for spin-echo sequences.

- Patients require patience. (It's important enough to repeat.)

BIBLIOGRAPHY

PRINCIPLES OF MRI

Brasch RC, ed. *MRI Contrast Enhancement in the Central Nervous System: A Case Study Approach.* New York: Raven Press; 1993.

Bushong SC. *Magnetic Resonance Imaging: Physical and Biological Principles.* St. Louis: Mosby-Year Book, Inc.; 1988.

Cardoza JD, Herfkens RJ. *MRI Survival Guide.* New York: Raven Press; 1994.

Falke TM, ed. *Essentials of Clinical MRI.* Boston: Nijhoff; 1988.

Friedman BR, et al. *Principles of MRI.* New York: McGraw-Hill; 1989.

Hendrick RE, Russ PD, Simon JH, eds. *MRI, Principles and Artifacts.* New York: Raven Press; 1993.

Knowles RJR. Principles of magnetic resonance imaging. In: Markisz JA, ed. *Musculoskeletal Imaging.* Boston: Little, Brown & Co.; 1991: 231–254.

Newhouse JH, Wiener JI. *Understanding MRI.* Boston: Little, Brown & Co.; 1991.

Oldendorf W, Oldendorf W, Jr. *MRI Primer.* New York: Raven Press; 1991.

Westbrook C. *Handbook of MRI Technique.* Cambridge, MA: Blackwell Scientific Publications; 1994.

Wolf GL, Popp C. *NMR: A Primer for Medical Imaging.* Thorofare, NJ: SLACK; 1984.

Young SW: *Magnetic Resonance Imaging: Basic Principles.* New York: Raven Press; 1988.

BIOLOGICAL EFFECTS AND SAFETY

Barber BJ, Schaefer DJ, Gordon CJ, Zawieja DC, Hecker J. Thermal effects of MR imaging: Worst-case studies on sheep. *Am J Roentgenol.* 1990; 155(5): 1105–1110.

Boutin RD, Briggs JE, Williamson MR. Injuries associated with MR imaging: Survey of safety records and methods used to screen patients for metallic foreign bodies before imaging. *Am J Roentgenol.* 1994; 162(1): 189–194.

Brown TR, Goldstein B, Little J. Severe burns resulting from magnetic resonance imaging with cardiopulmonary monitoring. Risks and relevant safety precautions. *Am J Phys Med Rehabil.* 1993; 72(3): 166–167.

DeLuca SA, Castronovo FP, Jr. Hazards of magnetic resonance imaging. *Am Fam Physician.* 1990; 41(1): 145–146.

Elster AD. Does MR imaging have any known effects on the developing fetus? *Am J Roentgenol.* 1994; 162(6): 1493.

Gleason CA, Kaula NF, Hricak H, Schmidt RA, Tanagho EA. The effect of magnetic resonance imagers on implanted neurostimulators. *Pacing Clin Electrophysiol.* 1992; 15(1): 81–94.

Kanal E, Shellock FG. The value of published data on MR compatibility of metallic implants and devices. *Am J Neuroradiol.* 1994; 15(7): 1394–1396.

Kanal E, Shellock FG, Talagala L. Safety considerations in MR imaging. *Radiology.* 1990; 176(3): 593–606.

Kelsey CA, King JN, Keck GM, Chiu MT, Wolfe DM, Orrison WW, Jr. Ocular hazard of metallic fragments during MR imaging at 0.06 T. *Radiology.* 1991; 180(1): 282–283.

Klucznik RP, Carrier DA, Pyka R, Haid RW. Placement of a ferromagnetic intracerebral aneurysm clip in a magnetic field with a fatal outcome. *Radiology.* 1993; 187(3): 855–856.

Kuethe DO, Small KW, Blinder RA, Non-ferromagnetic retinal tacks are a tolerable risk in magnetic resonance imaging. *Invest Radiol.* 1991; 26(1): 1–7.

LaBan MM, Viola S, Williams DA, Wang AM. Magnetic resonance imaging of the lumbar herniated disc in pregnancy. *Am J Phys Med Rehabil.* 1995; 74(1): 59–61.

Mishkin M. Metallic surgical clips and magnetic resonance imaging. *JAMA.* 1994; 271(23): 1886.

Portnoy WM, Mattucci K. Cochlear implants as a contraindication to magnetic resonance imaging. *Ann Otol Rhinol Laryngol.* 1991; 100(3): 195–197.

Prasad N, Wright DA, Ford JJ, Thornby JI. Safety of 4-T MR imaging: Study of effects on developing frog embryos. *Radiology.* 1990; 174(1): 251–253.

Rupp R, Ebraheim NA, Savolaine ER, Jackson WT. Magnetic resonance imaging evaluation of the spine with metal implants. General safety and superior imaging with titanium. *Spine.* 1993; 18(3): 379–385.

Shellock FG, Kanal E. *Magnetic Resonance Bioeffects, Safety, and Patient Management.* New York: Raven Press; 1994.

Shellock FG, Schatz CJ. Metallic otologic implants: in vitro assessment of ferromagnetism at 1.5 T. *Am J Neuroradiol.* 1991; 12(2): 279–281.

Vogl TJ, Paulus W, Fuchs A, Krafczyk S, Lissner J. Influence of magnetic resonance imaging on evoked potentials and nerve conduction velocities in humans. *Invest Radiol.* 1991; 26(5): 432–437.

Williamson MR, Espinosa MC, Boutin RD, Orrison WW, Jr, Hart BL, Kelsey CA. Metallic foreign bodies in the orbits of patients undergoing MR imaging: Prevalence and value of radiography and CT before MR. *Am J Roentgenol.* 1994; 162(4): 981–983.

QUALITY ASSURANCE

Hyde RJ, Ellis JH, Gardner EA, Zhang Y, Carson PL. MRI scanner variability studies using a semi-automated analysis system. *Magn Reson Imaging.* 1994; 12(7): 1089–1097.

Knowles RJR, Markisz JA. *Quality Assurance and Image Artifacts in Magnetic Resonance Imaging.* Boston: Little, Brown & Co.; 1988.

Lerski RA. Trial of modifications to Eurospin MRI test objects. *Magn Reson Imaging.* 1993; 11(6): 835–839.

Lerski RA, de Certaines JD. Performance assessment and quality control in MRI by Eurospin test objects and protocols. *Magn Reson Imaging.* 1993; 11(6): 817–833.

Moore CC, Reeder SB, McVeigh ER. Tagged MR imaging in a deforming phantom: Photographic validation. *Radiology.* 1994; 190(3): 765–769.

Murphy BW, Carson PL, Ellis JH, Zhang YT, Hyde RJ, Chenevert TL. Signal-to-noise measures for magnetic resonance imagers. *Magn Reson Imaging.* 1993; 11(3): 425–428.

Simmons A, Tofts PS, Barker GJ, Arridge SR. Sources of intensity nonuniformity in spin echo images at 1.5 T. *Magn Reson Med.* 1994; 32(1): 121–128.

IMAGE ARTIFACTS

Hendrick RE, Russ PD, Simon JH, eds. *MRI, Principles and Artifacts.* New York: Raven Press; 1993.

Knowles RJR, Markisz JA. *Quality Assurance and Image Artifacts in Magnetic Resonance Imaging.* Boston: Little, Brown & Co.; 1988.

PATIENT CARE

Avrahami E: Panic attacks during MR imaging: Treatment with i.v. diazepam. *Am J Neuroradiol.* 1990; 11(4): 833–835.

Brand KP. How well is your patient prepared for an MRI? An insider's perspective. *Cancer Nurs.* 1994; 17(6): 512–515.

Coulden RA, Dixon AK, Freer CE, Antoun NM, Moore NR, Sims C, Hall LD. Magnetic resonance imaging: When is one sequence sufficient? *Clin Radiol.* 1991; 44(6): 393–396.

Elster AD, Link KM, Carr JJ. Patient screening prior to MR imaging: A practical approach synthesized from protocols at 15 U. S. medical centers. *Am J Roentgenol.* 1994; 162(1): 195–199.

Katz RC, Wilson L, Frazer N. Anxiety and its determinants in patients undergoing magnetic resonance imaging. *J Behav Ther Exp Psychiatry.* 1994; 25(2): 131–134.

MacKenzie R, Sims C, Owens RG, Dixon AK. Patients' perceptions of magnetic resonance imaging. *Clin Radiol.* 1995; 50(3): 137–143.

Martin JB, Ahles TA, Jeffery R. The role of private body consciousness and anxiety in the report of somatic symptoms during magnetic resonance imaging. *J Behav Ther Exp Psychiatry.* 1991; 22(1):3–7.

McCauley TR, Wright JG, Bell SM, McCarthy S. Effect of prone versus supine patient positioning on pelvic magnetic resonance image quality. *Invest Radiol.* 1992; 27(12): 1005–1008.

Melendez JC, McCrank E. Anxiety-related reactions associated with magnetic resonance imaging examinations *JAMA.* 1993; 270(6): 745–747.

Och JG, Clarke GD, Sobol WT, Rosen CW, Mun SK. Acceptance testing of magnetic resonance imaging systems: Report of AAPM nuclear magnetic resonance task group no. 6. *Med Phys.* 1992; 19(1): 217–229.

Price RR, Axel L, Morgan T, Newman R, Perman W, Schneiders N, Selikson M, Wood M, Thomas SR. Quality assurance methods and phantoms for magnetic resonance imaging: Report of AAPM nuclear magnetic resonance task group no. 1. *Med Phys.* 1990; 17(2): 287–295.

Thorp D, Owens RG, Whitehouse G, Dewey ME. Subjective experiences of magnetic resonance imaging. *Clin Radiol.* 1990; 41(4): 276–278.

Wright JG, McCauley TR, Bell SM, McCarthy S. The reliability of radiologists' quality assessment of MR pelvic scans. *J Comput Assist Tomogr.* 1992; 16(4): 592–596.

ANATOMY

Clemente CH. *Anatomy: A Regional Atlas of the Human Body.* Baltimore: Urban & Schwarzenberg; 1981.

El-Khoury, GY, Bergman RA, Montgomery WJ. *Sectional Anatomy by MRI.* 2nd ed. New York: Churchill Livingstone; 1995.

Koritké JG, Sick H. *Atlas of Sectional Human Anatomy.* 2nd ed. Baltimore: Urban & Schwarzenberg; 1988.

Kucharczyk W, ed. *MRI: Central Nervous System.* New York: Lippincott; 1990.

Lufkin RB, Hanafee WN, eds. *MRI of the Head and Neck.* New York: Raven Press; 1991.

Markisz JA, ed. *Musculoskeletal Imaging: MRI, CT, Nuclear Medicine, and Ultrasound in Clinical Practice.* Boston: Little, Brown & Co.; 1991.

Markisz JA, Rafal RB, Kazam E. *MRI Atlas of the Pelvis: Normal Anatomy and Pathology.* Baltimore: Williams & Wilkins; 1993.

Markisz JA, Rafal RB, Kazam E. *MR Atlas of the Neck and Chest.* Cambridge, MA: Blackwell Scientific Publications; 1996.

Markisz JA, Ramirez E, Kazam E. *MR Atlas of the Abdomen.* Cambridge, MA: Blackwell Scientific Publications; 1996.

Wolpert SM, Barnes PD. *MRI in Pediatric Neuroradiology.* St. Louis: Mosby Year Book; 1992.

Zirinsky K, Markisz JA. *Cross-sectional Abdominal Anatomy: CT, MRI, and Ultrasound: A Programmed Atlas.* New York: Igaku-Shoin; 1992.

GLOSSARY

absolute zero: The lowest possible temperature that can be obtained. Called absolute zero, it occurs at –273.16°C, or –459.69°F, and is written as 0 K. The absolute zero temperature scale is also called the Kelvin scale, after William Thomson, a Scot who became Lord Kelvin in 1892, and developed the scale.

acquisition matrix: The number of pixels in the phase-encoding direction and the frequency-encoding direction.

acquisition time: The amount of time necessary to collect all of the data for a particular sequence.

active shielding: A magnetic shielding, which utilizes secondary coils that interact with the primary magnetic field to cancel or reduce the magnetic fringe field from around the magnet.

aliasing: A wrap-around artifact, caused by too small a field of view or too small an acquisition matrix in the phase-encoding direction. The tissue to the left of the imaged region appears superimposed on the right side.

angular frequency: A measure of the rate of rotation, with units of radians per second.

array coil: An rf coil composed of multiple smaller coils, which can be combined or used individually.

array coil, coupled: Array coils that are connected to each other through direct electrical linkage or by inductance.

array coil, isolated: Array coils that are electrically insulated from each other and have individual transmit and receive circuits. Data from these isolated coils is processed independently.

array coil, phased: Multiple small coils arranged to efficiently cover a specific anatomic region and obtain high-resolution, high-SNR images of a larger volume. The data from the individual coils is integrated by special software to produce the high-resolution images.

array processor: A component of the computer system designed to perform numerical calculations rapidly. It is necessary to speed up calculations for converting data to images.

artifact: Spurious information in an image, which can be due to a large number of causes, including motion, foreign objects, system failure, or computer processing.

atom: The smallest part of an element. It is composed of a nucleus, consisting of positively charged protons and neutral neutrons, surrounded by negatively charged electrons.

attenuation: A reduction in size. An attenuated signal refers to a signal that has been reduced in strength.

bandwidth: The range of frequencies contained in a signal. A bandwidth of 16 Khz would contain all frequencies from 8 KHz below the main frequency to 8 KHz above.

cardiac gating: Technique of synchronizing data acquisition with cardiac motion by triggering the rf pulse on the R wave of an ECG tracing.

chemical shift artifact: The appearance of a bright or dark line, at a fat–soft tissue interface due to the difference in resonant frequency (3 ppm) between fat protons and water protons (found in soft tissue structures).

coherence: The property of a set of waves or moving bodies in which the motions or oscillations maintain a definite and continuing fixed relationship to each other.

coil: A loop of metal devised to act as a receiver or transmitter of rf signal (surface coil); or to produce a small magnetic field to produce a change in the overall field strength at a given position (gradient coil).

contrast: The difference in signal intensities between two adjacent pixels.

contrast agent: A material furnished to produce a large change in signal intensities, usually by altering the T1 and/or T2 values of the affected tissues.

contrast-to-noise ratio: The difference in signal intensity between two points divided by the signal due to background noise.

cryogenic temperatures: An indefinite temperature range, which begins at approximately the boiling point of oxygen, 90°K (the high end of the range) down to near absolute zero (–459.69°F, –273.16°C, or 0°K). The boiling point of liquid helium is 4.2°K (–268.9°C, –452°F), and that of liquid nitrogen is 47.3°K (–195.8°C, –320.4°F). The theoretical limit for the lowest temperature possible is five ten-millionths of a degree above absolute zero (0.0000005°K).

cryogens: Refrigerants, usually liquid helium and/or liquid nitrogen, used to obtain and maintain cryogenic temperatures.

cryostat: A device used to maintain cryogenic temperatures.

decay: Decrease in signal due to a loss of transverse magnetization.

decibel: A numerical expression used to characterize the relative loudness of sounds. The decibel level of a sound is ten times the common logarithm (base 10) of the ratio of the power levels.

dephasing: Loss of phase coherence of transverse magnetization.

diamagnetic: The property that certain substances have of being weakly repelled by both poles of a magnet.

diffusion: Mixing of molecules due to their random motion.

digital-to-analog converter: Electronic unit that transforms digital signals into an analog (continuous) signal.

dipole: Any system having two equal but opposite electric charges or magnetic poles separated by a very small distance.

echo planar imaging: Rapid imaging method with high-speed gradient coils, which permits obtaining an entire image with one excitation pulse.

echo time: The time between the application of the excitation pulse and the appearance of the echo; abbreviated TE. In spin-echo imaging it is twice the time between the 90° excitation pulse and the 180° rephasing pulse.

echo train: The series of 180° rephasing pulses producing echoes during a fast spin-echo sequence.

eddy currents: Small electrical currents induced in an electrical conductor by changing magnetic fields. Eddy currents can then produce small local inhomogeneities in the overall magnetic field, which will produce image artifacts.

eddy current correction: Methods of decreasing the effects of eddy current inhomogeneities by modifying input or using shielded coils.

electromagnet: A soft iron core surrounded by a coil of wire, which temporarily becomes a magnet when an electric current flows through the wire.

electromagnetic energy: Energy produced by the electromagnetic waves that constitute the electromagnetic spectrum.

electromagnetic radiation: The electromagnetic waves that constitute the electromagnetic spectrum. Higher frequencies (higher energies) than visible light can be harmful, causing DNA and tissue damage.

electromagnetic spectrum: The complete range of frequencies of electromagnetic waves from the lowest to the highest, including, in order, radiowaves, infrared rays, visible light, ultraviolet rays, X-rays, and gamma rays.

electron: Smallest common subatomic particle, which has a negative charge. The movement of electrons through a wire is electricity.

energy: The ability to do work. Energy is found in many widely different forms: kinetic (motion), electrical, mechanical, heat, light, potential, etc.

equilibrium: A state of balance, during which no net changes occur.

ferromagnetic: A material, such as iron, nickel, or cobalt, having a high magnetic permeability that varies with the magnetizing force.

FID: Free induction decay.

field: A physical quantity specified at points throughout a region of space (e.g., the values of the magnetic field at various positions around the magnet as demonstrated in Figures 5.4, 5.5, and 5.6).

field homogeneity: Maintenance of a uniform magnetic field over the entire imaging volume.

field of view: The area covered by a scan.

flip angle: Radiofrequency energy produced by rf transmitter, which rotates the equilibrium magnetic vector through a specific angle.

force: Anything that produces, stops, or changes motion, and that, if unopposed, can push or pull objects.

Fourier transform: A complex mathematical technique, which changes the mathematical form of the data obtained during the imaging process into a more useful format so that images can be configured.

FOV: Field of view.

free induction decay: The decrease in longitudinal signal from a system after the rf pulse has been turned off.

frequency: The number of times per second a process repeats itself. The unit of frequency is hertz, where 1 Hz is one repetition per second.

frequency encoding: Assigning a discrete frequency to each pixel along the direction of the frequency-encoding axis by applying a magnetic gradient along the axis.

G: Abbreviation for **gauss.**

gadolinium: A rare-earth element with an atomic number of 64, found in the lanthanide series of the periodic table of the elements. Used as a trivalent ion, it is toxic to humans in its natural form, but when combined with a chelating agent it is safe to use for an intravenous magnetic contrast material.

gadolinium-DTPA: Gadolinium diethylenetriamine pentaacetic acid, the first gadolinium contrast agent approved by the FDA.

gating: A data-acquisition technique that minimizes the effects of physiologic motion by triggering the rf pulse on a physiologic signal (e.g., end inspiration, R wave of an ECG).

gauss: A unit of magnetic field strength, along with tesla; abbreviated G. 10,000 G = 1 T. The magnetic field of the Earth is approximately 0.5 G, varying from 0.7 G at the poles to 0.3 G at the equator.

gradient: The direction and rate of change of a quantity. A magnetic gradient placed along a line would change the strength of the magnetic field by a certain fixed amount at every point along the line.

gradient coils: Electromagnetic coils used to produce a uniform magnetic gradient along a particular direction (x axis, y axis, or z axis).

gradient echo: A signal (echo) produced by gradient changes to refocus the rf pulse, rather than a 180° refocusing rf pulse.

gradient echo imaging: A rapid imaging method that employs flip angles smaller than 90° and a gradient pulse to refocus the spins, rather than a 180° refocusing rf pulse.

gradient steps: The actual change in value from one level to another—for example, the differences in the magnetic gradient between each pair of successive slices in the slice-encoding direction. (See also **gradient.**)

gyromagnetic ratio: A physical constant, unique for each nucleus, defined as the ratio of the magnetic moment of the nucleus to its angular momentum. For the hydrogen nucleus it is equal to 42.58 MHz/T.

hertz: A unit of frequency, equal to one cycle per second.

hybrid magnet: A magnet composed of both resistive magnet components, along with a permanent magnet, to produce a magnetic field.

Hz: Abbreviation for **hertz,** a unit of frequency.

image acquisition time: The total time required for data acquisition during a pulse sequence. For spin-echo images this is equal (in seconds) to the product of the repetition time (TR), the number of excitations (N_{ex}), and the number of phase-encoding steps, divided by 1,000.

intensity: The relative strength of a signal: the amount of force or energy of heat, light, sound, magnetic flux, electric current, etc., per unit area or volume.

interpulse time: The time (usually in milliseconds) between the application of the various rf pulses during any given pulse sequence.

interslice thickness: The space between sections being imaged during a data acquisition sequence.

inversion recovery imaging: Method of imaging in which inversion recovery (IR) sequences produce heavily T1-weighted images by first applying a 180° pulse; then, after a time TI (inversion time), a 90° pulse; and finally a 180° refocusing pulse.

inversion time: The time between the center of the 180° rephasing (or inverting) pulse and the 90° excitation pulse during an inversion recovery sequence; abbreviated TI.

ionizing radiation: Potentially hazardous high-energy radiation that can cause ionization of molecules (breakup of molecules into ions), particularly DNA.

isocenter: The geometric center of the magnetic field within the bore of the magnet.

Kelvin: The unit of the absolute temperature scale. The Kelvin is named after its developer, Lord Kelvin of Scotland, one of the world's premier physicists, who published more than 650 scientific papers (12 before he was 21), held 70 patents, was president of the Royal Society, was knighted by Queen Victoria, and supervised the laying of the first trans-Atlantic cable in 1866.

KHz: Abbreviation for **kilohertz,** a unit of frequency.

kilohertz: A unit of frequency equal to 1,000 hertz, or 1,000 cycles per second.

K-space: An abstract concept used to explain how acquired data is stored in a hypothetical linear matrix.

Larmor equation: An equation stating that the frequency for nuclear magnetic resonance is equal to the product of the gyromagnetic ratio times the magnetic field strength.

Larmor frequency: Specific radiofrequency (rf) at which magnetic resonance occurs.

longitudinal relaxation time: The loss of longitudinal relaxation as the overall magnetic vector returns to $1/e$, or 63% of its initial value, as it realigns itself with the main magnetic field after the rf pulse has been turned off; also called T1 relaxation time.

magnet: Any material, such as iron, that has the property of attracting like material by producing a magnetic field.

magnetic dipole: A small magnet with north and south poles, created by spinning charges in the nucleus.

magnetic field: The region surrounding a magnet; a vector quantity that produces a magnetizing force on an object placed within it.

magnetic fringe field: The magnetic field outside of the bore of a magnet.

magnetic gradient: A small magnetic field used to produce changes in the overall magnetic field in a given direction.

magnetic moment: A vector quantity denoting the direction and size of the magnetic field associated with a particle.

magnetic resonance: A resonance phenomenon during which a particular frequency (Larmor frequency) will induce a transition from a lower energy state to a higher energy state.

magnetic resonance imaging: Utilization of the principles of magnetic resonance to produce an image.

magnetic susceptibility: The ability of a material to become magnetized.

magnetite: A black iron oxide, Fe_3O_4, an important iron ore: the major component of the magnetic ore called lodestone.

magnetization transfer: Selective excitation of only one type of nucleus in a multicomponent system, allowing significantly increased contrast.

matrix: A set of numbers or objects arranged in columns and rows. In an MR image this refers to the rows of pixels in the frequency-encoding direction and the columns of pixels in the phase-encoding direction.

megahertz: A unit of frequency equal to 1 million hertz, or 1 million cycles per second.

MHz: Abbreviation for **megahertz,** a unit of frequency.

mobile protons: Protons in a chemical compound that are free to rotate.

M_x: The component of the magnetic vector along the x axis.

M_{xy}: The transverse magnetization; the component of the magnetic vector in the xy plane.

M_y: The component of the magnetic vector along the y axis.

M_z: The longitudinal magnetization; the component of the magnetic vector along the z axis.

neutron: Electrically neutral, a fundamental particle of which the nucleus is composed.

N_{ex}:   Number of signal averages used in acquiring an image.

noise: Random and unpredictable signal obtained during image acquisition from extraneous sources.

nuclear magnetic resonance: Absorption of specific electromagnetic energy by magnetic nuclei, which subsequently emit the energy and revert to their original state.

nucleus: The central portion of an atom containing positively charged protons and uncharged neutrons. The nucleus makes up over 99.99% of the mass of an atom.

paramagnetic: A material having a magnetic permeability slightly greater than 1, which varies only slightly when placed in an applied magnetic field.

partial saturation: Repeatedly applied rf pulses with a repetition time (TR) shorter than the T1 value of the tissue.

partial volume effect: Decreased resolution due to using too large a slice thickness; the signals of two or more different tissues are averaged in one voxel.

passive shielding: Eliminating or reducing the magnetic fringe field by applying highly permeable materials to the surface of the magnet, while maintaining the uniformity of the magnetic field within the bore.

passive shimming: Shimming a magnet by placing pieces of iron or other ferromagnetic materials directly on the MRI system in order to produce a homogeneous field within the bore of the system.

permanent magnet: A substance that produces a magnetic field because it is a permanently magnetized material.

permeability: The ability of a material to concentrate a magnetic field, thereby decreasing its range.

phase: The location of a wave relative to its starting point, or to a comparable wave.

phase encoding: Identifying the voxels emitting MR signals by applying a pulsed magnetic gradient, which causes each voxel to have a different phase.

phase-encoding gradient: The magnetic gradient that is applied to produce a variation in phase within the voxels along a given direction.

phased array coil: Multiple small coils arranged to efficiently cover a specific anatomic region and obtain high-resolution, high-SNR images of a larger volume. The data from the individual coils is integrated by special software to produce the high-resolution images.

pixel: The smallest segment of an image. The resolution of an image cannot be greater than the pixel size; however, the resolution may be less than the pixel size.

precession: A circular rotation of the magnetic vector of a nucleus around the main magnetic axis, to describe a conical shaped path, as does a wobbling spinning top.

precessional frequency: The speed of a magnetic precession.

proton: Positively charged particle found in the nucleus of an atom; the source of all signal used in MR imaging.

proton density image: An image in which the TR and TE are selected so that the weighting factor is most dependent upon the density of protons in the tissues. Signal intensities are intermediate between T1- and T2-weighted images.

pulse: A burst of rf energy corresponding to the Larmor frequency produced by the rf transmitter.

pulse angle (flip angle):   RF energy produced by the rf transmitter, which rotates the equilibrium magnetic vector through a specific angle.

pulse sequence: The specific sequence of rf pulses designed to produce a particular type of image (e.g., T1-weighted, STIR, gradient echo, etc.).

quench: Loss of superconductivity, which will produce heat that can rapidly evaporate the liquid helium in the cryostat, producing huge amounts of helium gas that has the potential to displace all of the oxygen in the scanning room.

radiofrequency: Frequency of electromagnetic radiation of radiowaves, lying below the infrared light portion of the spectrum, between approximately 10 kHz and 1,000,000 MHz; abbreviated rf.

radiowaves: Low-energy, non-ionizing electromagnetic radiation with a frequency lying in the radiofrequency range.

relaxation time: The time that it takes for a system to revert to $1/e$ of its equilibrium value, which is approximately 63%.

repetition time: The time between successive excitation pulses; abbreviated TR.

resolution: The dimension of the smallest distinct object that can be visualized on an image.

resonance: The intensification that occurs when a small oscillation of an object is greatly increased by a periodic force (sound or electromagnetic energy wave) at the same or nearly the same frequency.

rf: Abbreviation for **radiofrequency.**

rf pulse: A pulse of electromagnetic energy in the radiofrequency range corresponding to the Larmor frequency, produced by the rf transmitter.

saturation: Nonequilibrium state with equal numbers of nuclei ordered with and against the overall magnetic field, caused by rapidly applied rf pulses. Material that has undergone saturation will not produce an MR signal.

shielding: Protection of or from the environment. Magnetic shielding is used to decrease the fringe field around the magnet; rf shielding is used to keep stray radiofrequencies from entering the scanning room.

shim coils: Electrical coils used to produce small magnetic fields to correct for field inhomogeneity.

shimming: The process of correcting magnetic fields for areas of nonhomogeneity, either by applying ferromagnetic materials to the magnet (passive shimming) or by using electrical coils to produce a magnetic field to counteract the inhomogeneities.

signal average: Average of several different data acquisitions for the same pixel in order to counteract the effect of noise or artifacts.

signal decay: Loss of signal over time due to decrease in transverse magnetization.

signal-to-noise ratio: The ratio of the signal intensity divided by the noise.

slice-encoding gradient: The magnetic gradient that is applied to determine the position of the anatomic section to be imaged.

slice thickness: The thickness of the anatomic section being imaged, which is also the depth of each voxel.

SNR: Signal-to-noise ratio, the value of the signal intensity from a tissue divided by the signal from the background, in which there is no tissue.

spin echo: The appearance of an rf signal from a system that has undergone dephasing, by rephasing or refocusing the signal by a 180° pulse.

spin-echo imaging: The most popular pulse sequence, which employs a 90° excitation pulse followed by a 180° refocusing pulse.

superconducting magnet: High-field magnets that employ the principles of superconducting metals to produce a magnetic field.

superconductivity: When certain metals and alloys are cooled to very low temperatures they essentially achieve an absence of all electrical resistance; first discovered in 1911 by Heike Kamerlingh Onnes. MRI systems using this principle can produce high field strengths.

surface coil: A small coil, usually shaped to fit the part of the body being imaged, which can be either a receive coil or a transmit/receive coil. It produces high-resolution images of a small portion of the anatomy.

T: Abbreviation for **tesla;** unit of magnetic field strength.

T1:   A measure of the time necessary for a magnetic vector that has been tipped away from the direction of the main magnetic field to return to $1/e$, or 63% of its equilibrium value.

T1 relaxation time: Longitudinal relaxation time. Loss of longitudinal relaxation as the overall magnetic vector realigns itself with the main magnetic field after the rf pulse has been turned off.

T1-weighted image: An image produced with a short TR and a short TE, so that the contribution from the T1 value of the tissue is much more important than the T2 contribution. These images usually have very high resolution but decreased tissue contrast.

T2:   A measure of the time necessary for the loss of transverse magnetization due to spin-spin relaxation; the time it takes for a 63% decrease in transverse relaxation time.

T2 relaxation time: Transverse relaxation time. The decrease of phase coherence leading to a decrease in the transverse magnetization due to spin-spin relaxation.

T2-weighted image: An image produced with a long TR and a long TE, so that the contribution from the T1 value of the tissue is much less important than the T2 contribution. These images usually have diminished resolution but markedly increased contrast.

T2*:   Dephasing of spins caused by local magnetic inhomogeneities due to local susceptibility differences, motion of flowing spins, and field variations.

TE: Echo time: the time between the excitation pulse and the detection of the echo signal. In spin-echo imaging it is equal to twice the time between the 90° excitation pulse and the 180° rephasing pulse.

tesla: Unit of magnetic field strength (flux density); 10,000 G is equal to one tesla (T).

TI: Inversion time.

TR: Repetition time.

transverse relaxation time: The decrease of phase coherence leading to a decrease in the transverse magnetization due to spin-spin relaxation (T2).

voxel: A volume equal to the area of the pixel times the thickness of the slice for a given image. The total signal produced from within the voxel determines the appearance of the pixel.

ABBREVIATIONS AND ACRONYMS

In an unfortunate trend, most manufacturers have resorted to the use of acronyms to describe different pulse sequences or imaging options used on their equipment during the imaging process. While the use of acronyms does shorten both written and verbal references to complex terms, this tendency has caused an immense amount of confusion when users of products from two different manufactures attempt to communicate. Is MAST equivalent to SMART? What about PEAR and FREEZE, or GRASS and GRECO? We find that these acronyms have created a language barrier between users of different brands of MR units. We have listed some of the acronyms used by different manufactures, along with their official descriptions and a general categorization of what they do.

Acronym	Description	Classification
3D MP-RAGE	three-dimensional magnetization prepared rapid gradient echo	T1-weighted gradient echo
BFAST	blood flow artifact suppression technique	saturation pulse
CE-FAST	contrast-enhanced FAST	gradient echo
CFAST	cerebrospinal fluid artifact suppression technique	motion artifact reduction

(continued)

Acronym	Description	Classification
ChemSat	chemical saturation	saturation pulse
DE FGR	driven equilibrium fast GRASS	gradient echo
DFSE	dual-echo fast spin echo	fast spin echo
E-SHORT	short repetition technique	gradient echo
F-SHORT	short repetition technique based on free induction decay	gradient echo
FAST	Fourier acquired steady-state technique	gradient echo
FATSAT	fat saturation	saturation pulse
FC	glow compensation	motion artifact reduction
FE	field echo	gradient echo
FFE	fast field echo	gradient echo
FGR	fast GRASS	gradient echo
FISP	fast imaging with steady-state precession	gradient echo
FLAG	flow-adjustable gradients	motion artifact reduction
FLAIR	fluid attenuated inversion recovery	inversion recovery
FLASH	fast low-angle shot	T1-weighted gradient echo
FLOWCOMP	flow compensation	motion artifact reduction
FREEZE	respiratory selection of phase-encoding steps	respiratory compensation
FSE	fast spin echo	fast spin echo
FSPE	respiratory sorted phase encoding	respiratory compensation
FSPGR	fast SPGR	T1-weighted gradient echo
GE	gradient echo	gradient echo
GFE	gradient field echo	gradient echo
GFEC	gradient field echo with contrast	gradient echo
GMC	gradient moment compensation	motion artifact reduction
GMN	gradient moment nulling	motion artifact reduction
GMR	gradient moment rephasing	motion artifact reduction
GR	gradient rephasing	motion artifact reduction
GRASS	gradient-recalled acquisition in steady state	gradient echo
GRE	gradient-recalled echo	gradient echo
GRE	gradient rephasing	motion artifact reduction

(continued)

Acronym	Description	Classification
GRECO	gradient-recalled echo	gradient echo
IR FGR	inversion recovery fast GRASS	T1-weighted gradient echo
MAST	motion artifact suppression technique	motion artifact reduction
MEMS	multi-echo multi-shot	fast spin echo
MESS	multi-echo single shot	fast spin echo
MOTSA	multiple overlapping thick slab angiography	MRA technique
MPGR	multiplanar gradient recalled	gradient echo
PEAR	phase-encoded artifact reduction	respiratory compensation
Phase Reordering	phase reordering	respiratory compensation
PRE-SAT	presaturation technique	saturation pulse
PRESAT	presaturation	saturation pulse
PRI	partial flip imaging	gradient echo
PSIF	reverse FISP	gradient echo
RARE	rapid acquisition with relaxation enhancement	fast spin echo
RESCOMP	respiratory compensation	respiratory compensation
REST	regional saturation	saturation pulse
RF Spoiled FAST	RF-spoiled Fourier acquired steady-state technique	T1-weighted gradient echo
RISE	rapid imaging spin echo	fast spin echo
ROAST	resonant offset averaging in the steady state	gradient echo
SAT	saturation	saturation pulse
SATURATION	selectable presaturation	saturation pulse
SMART	Shimadzu motion artifact reduction technique	motion artifact reduction
SMASH	short-repetition techniques	gradient echo
SPGR	spoiled gradient recalled	T1-weighted gradient echo
SPIR	spectral presaturation with inversion recovery	saturation pulse
SSFP	steady-state free precession	gradient echo
STAGE	small tip-angle gradient echo	gradient echo
STAGE-T1W	small tip angle gradient echo: T1 weighted	T1-weighted gradient echo

(continued)

Acronym	Description	Classification
STERF	steady-state technique with refocused free induction decay	
STILL	flow and motion compensation	motion artifact reduction
STIR	short T1 inversion recovery	fat saturation IR
T1-FFE	contrast enhanced fast field echo	T1-weighted gradient echo
T2-FFE	contrast enhanced fast field echo	gradient echo
TFE	turbo field echo	gradient echo
True-FISP	FIST with heavy T2 weighting	gradient echo
TSE	turbo spin echo	fast spin echo
TurboFLASH	magnetization prepared subsecond imaging technique	gradient echo

INDEX

A

Active shielding, 72
Air, as a contrast agent, 146
Alarms, for oxygen levels, 179
Aliasing, 201–5. *See also*
    Wrap-around
Alignment of atoms, 32, 32*f*,
    33*f*, 34*f*, 39*f*
Amplifiers
   artifacts and, 201
   gradient, 77–78
   rf, 79, 201
Analog-to-digital converter
    (ADC), 79
Appointments for patients, 235
Archiving, 68*f*, 225–28
   hardware and software for,
     225–26
   labeling and cataloging in,
     227–28
   media for, 226–27
Arteriovenous malformation,
    phase-contrast
    angiogram of, 106, 107*f*
Artifacts, 75, 183–217
   aliasing and, 201–5
   avoidance of, 212

drop-bit, 201
categories of, 183–84
eddy currents and, 78
eliminating (pruning) empty
    image space and,
    154–58, 154*f*, 155–56*f*,
    157*f*
ferromagnetic compounds
    and, 177, 191, 191*f*
flow compensation for,
    149–50, 152*f*
flowing blood appearance
    and, 192, 194–97
ghosting, 149, 192–94,
    199
gradients, 199–201
gradient instabilities and,
    199–201, 202–3*f*
image blurring with ringed
    structures and, 192–94,
    192–93*f*
imaging process and, 201–12,
    216–17*t*
implants and, 185–87
instrumental effects and,
    199–201, 216–17*t*
leaks in rf shielding and,
    82, 83*f*

Page numbers followed by *t* and *f* refer to
table and figures, respectively.

Page numbers followed by *t* and *f* refer to
table and figures, respectively.

E

Earplugs, 169
Echo, 64
Echo time (TE)
  different echo and, 89, 93*f*
  fast spin-echo imaging and,
    94, 249–50
  flow compensation and, 150
  pulse sequence and, 89
  radiofrequency (rf) signal
    and, 64
  scanning parameters affected
    by, 111, 120, 121–25
  signal-to-noise ratio (SNR)
    and, 120–25, 122*f*, 123*f*,
    124*f*, 125*f*
  spin-echo imaging and,
    87–88, 88*f*, 90*f*–91*f*
Echo train, in fast spin-echo
    imaging, 92
Eddy currents, 78
Elbow prostheses, 176
Electric current
  electromagnets and, 8
  superconductivity and, 8, 9
Electrical burns, and safety
    precautions, 177–78
Electrocardiogram (ECG)
    gating, 129–36, 130*f*,
    131*f*, 194, 197
Electrocardiogram (ECG) leads,
    177–78
Electromagnetic energy, 36
Electromagnetic radiation,
    36–37
  spectrum of, 36*t*
Electromagnets, 8, 67, 68–69
Electrons, magnetic properties
    of, 2
Electron spin resonance, 12

Excitations, number of, 112
Examination time, 23–24
Excitation pulse, 53
Eyeliner dyes, 177, 191

F

Faraday, Michael, 8
Fast spin echo (FSE) imaging,
    93–94, 138, 249–50
Fat
  artifacts in soft tissue
    imaging and, 207–10
  saturation techniques for,
    142, 145, 145*f*
  short TI inversion recovery
    (STIR) imaging and,
    95–96
Ferromagnetic materials
  artifacts from, 177, 191, 191*f*
  as contrast agents, 146, 149
  magnetic properties of, 5, 6, 6*f*
Field of view (FOV)
  artifacts and, 152
  eliminating (pruning) empty
    image space and,
    154–58, 154*f*, 155–56*f*,
    157*f*
  fractional, 156, 157*f*
  imaging time and, 244*t*, 249
  offset, 156, 157*f*
  scanning parameters affected
    by, 111, 113, 126*t*
Field strength, and signal-to-
    noise ratio (SNR), 29
Film, 229
Filters, 204
Flip angle, 54, 55*f*, 89, 111
Flow compensation, 102, 106,
    149–51, 152*f*

Page numbers followed by *t* and *f* refer to
table and figures, respectively.

Page numbers followed by *t* and *f* refer to
table and figures, respectively.

Page numbers followed by *t* and *f* refer to
table and figures, respectively.